Regulation
and
UK Optometry

Regulation
and
UK Optometry

Steve Taylor

Stephen Taylor Associates, UK

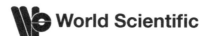

NEW JERSEY · LONDON · SINGAPORE · BEIJING · SHANGHAI · HONG KONG · TAIPEI · CHENNAI · TOKYO

Published by

World Scientific Publishing Co. Pte. Ltd.

5 Toh Tuck Link, Singapore 596224

USA office: 27 Warren Street, Suite 401-402, Hackensack, NJ 07601

UK office: 57 Shelton Street, Covent Garden, London WC2H 9HE

British Library Cataloguing-in-Publication Data
A catalogue record for this book is available from the British Library.

REGULATION AND UK OPTOMETRY

ISBN 978-981-126-144-2 (hardcover)
ISBN 978-981-126-215-9 (paperback)
ISBN 978-981-126-145-9 (ebook for institutions)
ISBN 978-981-126-146-6 (ebook for individuals)

For any available supplementary material, please visit
https://www.worldscientific.com/worldscibooks/10.1142/12998#t=suppl

Typeset by Stallion Press
Email: enquiries@stallionpress.com

Printed in Singapore

Disclaimer

The author has made every attempt to ensure that the content of the text is both accurate and current, however as mentioned in the introduction temporary changes have been introduced in response to the Covid pandemic of 2020 that may become permanent but that are not included in this text also there will be continuing regulatory and interpretive developments that mean the text can only be a guide to what is correct at any single moment in time. The text therefore should be used as a reference source to help to direct the reader, but then should the need arise it is essential that legal advice or the advice of professional bodies is sought and neither the author or the publisher take responsibility for actions taken or outcomes based on the content of this text.

Acknowledgements

Inevitably the writing of any text is dependent on the goodwill, time, support, and patience of many people. I would like to thank Joy at WSPC for her patience, the General Optical Council, and the College of Optometrists for permission to reproduce items, Harjit and the Federation of Ophthalmic and Dispensing Opticians for support in the publication process and my son Dean for help with cover design images. Most of all however my thanks must go to my wife Lorraine for demonstrating all the above characteristics and without her additional gentle nudging the text is unlikely to have appeared.

Optometrists in the United Kingdom are regulated by the General Optical Council. From oversight of optometric education and training, both at undergraduate and postgraduate level, to the conduct of clinical or disciplinary fitness-to-practice processes, the GOC plays an important role to ensure that primary eye care remains safe and fit for purpose. Understanding how regulatory processes work, how they have evolved, and how they may be changing in the future is of interest to all who care about the future of the eye care professions. Steve Taylor, a past president of the College of Optometrists, professional adviser to FODO and optometry adviser to NHS England and has been involved in the setting up of several undergraduate optometry programmes as an independent consultant. His text on the regulation of optometry in the UK will become a useful resource for optometrists and those who aim to join the profession. It will also fill an important gap for those who seek specific information on the evolution of UK optometry and its professional regulation.

Paul H Artes, PhD MCOptom
Professor in Eye & Vision Sciences
Faculty of Health: Medicine, Dentistry, and Human Sciences
University of Plymouth

This unique text provides a comprehensive guide to the regulatory framework for optometry in the UK. It is an essential companion for students of optometry and their supervisors as well as employers and practising clinicians. Steve Taylor has extensive experience across the sector, including in hospital and high street practice, education, industry and professional and regulatory bodies.

Yvonne Norgett
Senior Lecturer, <u>Faculty of Science and Engineering</u>
Anglia Ruskin University, Cambridge

Steve Taylor has been involved in optometry education, politics and regulation in the UK for 50 years and I look forward to seeing this text that will fill a gap on the optometry bookshelf.

Bob Hutchinson
Principal, Eros Business Consulting
CEO/Editor Opchat News
Past President of Royal Soc Medicine Primary Care Section

Contents

Introduction

The eyes and the law have been intimately connected since the time of Hammurabi.

Probably the most quoted and best-known legal phrase is a paraphrased translation of Hammurabi's code of ethics 'an eye for an eye and a tooth for a tooth'. As Hammurabi has been taken as the father of the legal system, then the eyes were, even in his days, considered important enough to be included at the birth.

The importance of the eye in society has maintained its high status. The early practitioners of ocular health ran a very great risk of loss of limb and financial ruin. In the Greek codes of law, a practitioner would lose his hands if he were to treat a nobleman and cause the loss of an eye. Should the eye belong to a servant, then the practitioner was expected to replace the servant if the treatment resulted in the loss of an eye. In view of the state of understanding (or lack of it) of surgery and intra-ocular disorders, and the inability to see into the eye before commencing treatment, it is surprising that anyone ventured into the risky business of eyecare. The advent of modern techniques and changes in the legal system have obviously helped to produce a healthier number of optical specialists with both hands intact!

The optical profession in Europe, as separate from the professions of medicine and ophthalmology, can obviously be traced back to the invention of spectacles. It is difficult to put a date on this as the initial years of spectacle production are shrouded in mystery. Marco Polo, reporting on his travels in China in 1275, mentioned that people wore glasses before their eyes for reading. The first evidence of the development of spectacles in Europe dates their invention to about AD 1280. Documents still exist in Venice, however, which refer to the manufacture of a form of spectacles which appeared in the first half of the thirteenth century. This evidence contradicts the general theory that a Florentinian, Salvino Degli Armati, was the inventor. He was credited with the invention in an inscription said to exist in a tomb in the church of Santa Maria Maggiore:

> Here lies Salvino Degli Armati son of Armato of Florence inventor of eyeglasses. May God forgive his sins. AD 1317.

The tomb is no longer in existence, and recent research has cast doubt upon the validity of the inscription.

It would seem that spectacles were in use by 1282, when a reference in the records of the Abbey of Saint Bavon le Grand indicates that a priest called Nicholas Bullett used spectacles when signing an agreement. It may be, however, that spectacles were reinvented by a Dominican monk who kept the invention a secret for commercial reasons. The evidence to support this comes from a reference in the Lenten Sermon on 23 February 1305 in the church of Santa Maria Novella in Florence. The sermon was given by Giordarno de Rivalto, who credited Friar Della Spina with the invention.

As a legal body, spectacle makers in Europe were first introduced into a Guild by Louis Xl of France in 1465. At this time the Guild also included haberdashers and upholsterers. This was changed in 1581 when Henry Ill granted a new guild consisting of mirror makers, toy makers and spectacle makers. The first German Guild of spectacle makers was established in Nuremberg in 1577. The Guild had the function of maintaining law and order within its profession.

In Britain the spectacle makers were incorporated by a Royal Charter granted by Charles I on 16 May 1629. The Charter, giving permission to form the Spectacle Makers Company, provided the opportunity to create laws and to produce a profession. It became a 'closed shop', with the Company granting only certain people, who had trained for their craft, permission to practise their trade. The original Charter gave the Court of the Spectacle Makers the power to make 'laws and statutes, decrees, ordinances and constitutions for the good rule and government of the Fellowship and craft'.

The Spectacle Makers Company began to lose a little control in the late 1800s, and the British Optical Association was eventually formed as an organised body in 1895. The function of the BOA was to improve standards within the profession, and an examination system was quickly established. Not to be outdone, the Spectacle Makers introduced their own examinations in 1898. The Spectacle Makers Company examinations at this time were mainly practical and biased towards the manufacture of lenses and frame materials. Sight testing was not incorporated into the examination syllabus until 1904.

Since these early days of the formation of the nucleus of a profession there has been a rapid rise in the standards of education and a requirement for registration. More recently the professional bodies have been rationalised to form a single examining body for optometry — the British College of Optometrists. Further development and cooperation between professionals were called for by the General Optical Council following the Optical Services Audit Committee report. On the consumer side, greater awareness of the services available, easier access of information through the internet and a better understanding of legal rights have led to a more demanding patient.

To meet these changes and potential developments with information technology several legislative orders have been introduced. The advances in the law relating to ocular health that are directly relevant to today's practising optometrist will be outlined in the chapters that follow.

As far as the optometrist is concerned there are two main sources of legal circumstance that can potentially affect them in their professional role. The first is action under common law and the second action under legislation. While the consequences and procedures for the two types may be very similar the development of the two legal situations has been very different.

Common Law

This can trace its roots back to the Middle Ages when the Normans through their system of feudal land tenure introduced a central government and laws common to all parts of England and later Wales. Under the system all land belonged absolutely to the Crown and persons holding land did so merely as tenants of the Crown. The Crown therefore had absolute powers over how the land and its occupants were treated. Consistency in legal matters was maintained by itinerant Royal judges who, in the King's name, travelled to all parts of the country settling disputes which related mainly to the possession of land. Gradually these judges were called upon to extend their jurisdiction to criminal matters and were able to lay the foundation of a Common Law of property and crime.

By the 13th century several changes to the system had steadied the development of Common Law. These changes mainly were instigated through the Barons who were protecting their self-interests by attempting to reduce the powers of the Royal Court in favour of their own profitable feudal courts that had been set up. Restrictions imposed by the Barons meant that Common Law continued to develop but along very conservative lines. One of the developments was for Common Law to expand from just criminal and property matters to include Law of Contract and Law of Tort. These two additions were to deal with civil wrongs that did not amount to a criminal offence.

By the Middle Ages four main types of Court had evolved:

1. Communal Courts applying local customary law. These declined as Common Law developed.
2. Seignorial Courts operated by the feudal landlords for their tenants. These also declined as Common Law developed.
3. Ecclesiastical Courts dealing with discipline of the clergy and matrimonial and testamentary matters. These courts declined after the Reformation and matrimonial and testamentary jurisdiction moved to the High Court in the 19th Century.
4. Royal Courts which included courts of Common Law and Equity. Within this umbrella several specialist areas were developed:

- The Courts of Assize dealing with criminal matters
- The Court of the King's Bench dealing with both criminal and civil actions involving the Crown
- The Court of Common Pleas dealing with civil action between subjects particularly relating to land
- The Court of Exchequer dealing with revenue matters
- The Court of Exchequer Chamber dealing with appeals from other Common Law courts

In the 19th Century Parliament made extensive reforms to the judicial system and administration of the law that ended many of the anachronisms in Common Law. By combining the administration of Common Law with that of Equity the Judicature Acts from 1873-1875 removed a final source of inconsistency and conflict.

Common Law is still the basis of modern English law and continues to develop by the Doctrine of Precedent by which judges apply established or customary rules of law to new cases as they arise. It is said to be "unwritten law" because there is no comprehensive set of statutes, judgements etc. that may be applied in a particular case.

Regulation and guidance in UK Optometry Regulation

Legislation is formed by regulations laid down by a body constituted for the purpose, such as the UK Parliament. Enacted laws of this type are called statutes. Legislation may be direct (e.g., Acts of Parliament) or indirect or delegated such as Statutory Instruments laid down by a Minister of the Government under power given by Act of Parliament. Currently UK Parliament is normally the supreme legislative body in the UK although in certain areas aspects of health legislation have been devolved down to national assemblies and in some situations despite the UKs exit from the European Union decisions may rest with the European Parliament. Delegated legislation is as binding as Parliamentary legislation. There is a general legislative clause however where it is considered that if anyone with delegated authority has exceeded their powers the laws laid down can be considered as void. This is the doctrine of ultra vires and has on occasions formed the basis of discussion within optometry.

Parliament consists of three essential components:

The Sovereign
The House of Lords
The House of Commons

Proposals for legislation must be placed before both Houses in the form of Bills. If approved by both Houses a Bill is then placed before the Sovereign for Royal Assent at which point the Bill becomes an Act of Parliament.

There is a difference between the legal systems in England, Wales, Scotland, and Northern Ireland all of which have their own Courts and their own National Assemblies able to make their own legislation covering certain aspects.

The need for delegated or subordinate legislation has increased as the time constraints on Parliament have been tightened and greater and greater technical knowledge is required in some areas to provide the fullest debate. The General Optical Council can therefore provide specialist expertise to delegated legislation proposed by the Minister for Health and is called upon from time to time to make comments or even to draft Statutory Instruments.

There are several legal systems with which the practitioner may come into contact besides criminal and civil actions. The Privy Council, which at one time wielded most of the governmental powers, is now largely formal and advisory in function. It is composed mainly of cabinet ministers, former ministers and Law Lords and led by a member of the Cabinet. It is a source of delegated legislation in the form of Orders in Council that may affect practice.

Administrative Tribunals associated with the Health Service are part of the complaints' procedure. If a complaint concerning a practitioner failing to comply with NHS Terms of Service were to be considered serious enough and could not be resolved informally then it would be referred to an Administrative Tribunal. The powers of such a Tribunal are restricted and ultimate decision, on appeal, lies with the Secretary of State.

The General Optical Council would fall within the classification of a Domestic Tribunal whose function is to maintain discipline/standards among members of a profession and to protect the public. Its role was established by the Opticians Act 1958 (revised and updated 1989), and it has delegated powers to make regulations in certain specified areas. The Privy Council does have power of veto and did use these powers during debate on changes to the contact lens regulations in 1984/85. The GOC however acts to maintain standards of practice in accordance with the duties laid down in the Opticians Act 1989. It has the power to remove a practitioner name from the register effectively preventing them from calling themselves an optometrist and therefore from sight testing.

The development of devolved powers to the individual countries within the UK to make regulation relating to health care has led to some significant differences to the provision of NHS services and although these are not included in detail, they are discussed briefly in Chapter 1. However, the fundamental general regulation of the profession of Optometry remains controlled through the UK Parliament and the General Optical Council.

Guidance

It is important to distinguish between regulation and guidance but also to remember that the GOC will take into account any available guidance when determining fitness to practise. The College of Optometrists for example has no statutory function but is effectively an organisation of members of the profession that offers guidance on good practice for the public benefit and the GOC will consider this as appropriate. Also as part of the regulation around registration the examination functions of the College of Optometrists are carried out on behalf of the GOC who regularly satisfy themselves that adequate standards are being met. As with any organisation there are agreed rules for College members and failure to comply may result in an individual's membership of the organisation being withdrawn. Unlike the consequences of removal from the GOC register, leaving the College will not prevent a practitioner from being registered and testing sight.

Other professional bodies such as ABDO, AOP and FODO are member organisations and again have no statutory function but may act against members with the ultimate sanction of removing membership. This action again does not prevent the individual from continuing to practise as long as they remain registered with the GOC.

2020 Coronavirus impact

The world pandemic of coronavirus that appeared in 2020 has had the consequence of requiring temporary legislation changes in the UK to take account of isolation and protective measures for operating face to face clinics. It has also seen temporary changes to the way that both the NHS and the GOC operate and the expectations of how care should be provided and continuing professional development/continuing education and training can be provided. As these have been introduced as temporary measures they are not discussed in this text although it is likely that some of the measures may well be retained once the pandemic allows some degree of return to normality in clinical settings for example the use of electronic conferencing for registrants to earn their CPD points has become accepted as normal.

Chapter 1

The National Health Service

Introduction

Since the acceptance by Parliament in 1946 of the ideals of a Health Service for all within the community, optometry has had a role. Initially that role was seen as being 'supplementary' to the Hospital Eye Service. Gradually, however, as it became clear that the Hospital Eye Service was never going to reach a point where it would be able to satisfy the demand for eye care, optometrists were included as part of the "General Ophthalmic Services" (GOS). Essentially individual optometrists, through Health Authorities, entered into a contract with the National Health Service to provide eye care, to those eligible, for a negotiated fee paid by the State. At the outset, this service was provided without charge to all patients, but over time this changed and currently eligibility for sight testing under GOS (and appliance supply) in England is restricted to specific groups of patients.

The development of the National Health Service has played a major role in the changes seen within optometry. Some would say that the link with the NHS has stifled the development of an adequately funded "eye examination" service and placed optometry in the situation in which it finds itself today, largely unappreciated for the eye care provided although this appears to be changing following the COVID pandemic of 2020/21. Others identify that in the initial stages of the NHS the funding available enabled the profession to become established and to concentrate on developing sight testing without the commercial pressures of today's environment. Whatever the truth of the matter, optometry and the National Health Service are less interwoven now than at any time since the 1946 Act.

Establishment of the National Health Service

On 6 November 1946, the National Health Service Act 1946 was passed by Parliament with the intention of establishing a comprehensive health service for England and Wales. According to the new Act it was the:

> '.... *duty of the Minister of Health ... to promote the establishment in England and Wales of a comprehensive health service designed to secure improvement in the physical and mental health of the people of England and Wales and the prevention, diagnosis and treatment of illness, and for that purpose to provide or secure the effective provision of services in accordance with the following provisions of the Act.'*

The National Health Service Act 1946 was set up according to four principles:

1   The health service should be financed by taxes and contributions paid when people were well rather than by charges levied on them when they were sick; and the financial burden of sickness should be spread over the whole community.
2   The health service should be truly national, aiming at providing the same high quality of service in every part of the country.
3   The service should provide full clinical freedom to the doctors working within it.
4   The health service should be centred upon the family doctor team providing the essential continuity to the health care of each individual and family, and mobilizing the services needed.

Since the National Health Service Act 1946, the following further relevant legislation has been enacted:

National Health Service (Scotland) Act 1947
Health Services Act (Northern Ireland) 1948
National Health Service (Amendment) Act 1949
National Health Service Act 1951
National Health Service Act 1952
National Health Service Act 1961
Health Services and Public Health Act 1968
National Health Service Re-Organisation Act 1973
National Health Service Act 1977
Health Services Act 1980
Health and Social Security Act 1984
Health and Medicines Act 1988
Opticians Act 1989
NHS and Community Care Act 1990
Health Authorities Act 1995
NHS (Primary Care) Act 1997
Health Act 1999
Health and Social Care Act 2001
NHS Reform and Health Care Professions Act 2002
NHS Act 2006
NHS Consequential Provisions Act 2006
Health Act 2006
Health and Social Care Act 2008
Health Act 2009
Health and Social Care Act 2012
Health and Care Act 2022

The gradual changes brought about by these Acts have produced a present-day situation that bears only a slight resemblance to that originally proposed. The changes can be demonstrated by a rapid but not exhaustive review of the intended impact of principal Acts.

National Health Service Act 1946

Under the original 1946 enactment the administration of the health service was divided into four main branches:

1. The Minister, as central planner, and co-ordinator would oversee each of the other branches and plan to integrate these as a whole and would also accept ultimate responsibility for the services.
2. The hospital and specialist services were to be administered on a regional basis by hospital boards, the exception being the teaching hospitals. To ensure maximum efficiency, the hospitals were further divided into local groups managed by hospital management committees.
3. Domiciliary care (not treatment) was to be provided by the Local Authorities and included:
    (a) the care of expectant mothers and young children;
    (b) domiciliary midwifery;
    (c) home nursing and health visiting;
    (d) vaccination and immunization;
    (e)   ambulance services and health centres;
    (f) the care of physically and mentally handicapped.
4. The general practitioner services were to be administered by the executive councils established under Part IV of the National Health Service Act 1946, s.31. Normally the executive councils were to be responsible for the services in the area of a local health authority, ensuring that there were sufficient practitioners within their area and administering the remuneration and terms and conditions of service.

To assist the Minister and to give advice on general matters relating to the administration of the health services a Central Health Services Council was established. In a further effort to maximize efficiency the Minister had the right to constitute standing advisory committees to provide specialist information on any specific aspects of the health services as and when it was required. These advisory committees fell into nine groups:

*   Standing Medical Advisory Committee.
*   Standing Dental Advisory Committee.
*   Standing Pharmaceutical Advisory Committee.
*   Standing Ophthalmic Advisory Committee.
*   Standing Nursing Advisory Committee.

- Standing Maternity and Midwifery Advisory Committee.
- Standing Mental Health Advisory Committee.
- Standing Tuberculosis Advisory Committee.
- Standing Council and Radiotherapy Advisory Committee.

This, then, provided a sound central administration with the ability to examine carefully any specialist problems that might arise.

In the case of the executive councils, a specialist knowledge was even more readily available. The 25 members of an executive council included: seven members appointed by the local medical committee, three members appointed by the local dental committee and two members appointed by the local pharmaceutical committee.

The local representative committees were formed where the Minister was satisfied that for the areas of any executive council, the committees were representative of:

- the medical practitioners of the area
- the dental practitioners of the area
- the people providing pharmaceutical services in the area.

Representatives of the optometrists and dispensing opticians providing supplementary ophthalmic services in the area were not formally recognized until the 1949 Act. Despite the recognition shown by the Act, ophthalmic membership of an executive council was not forthcoming until the Health Services and Public Health Act of 1968.

Role of the Minister of Health

Under the terms of the National Health Service Act 1946, the Minister was given the ultimate responsibility for the health service and was seen as the co-ordinator. The responsibilities and the position of the Minister could be summarized as follows:

- Central controller and planner, basing decisions on the information from the Central Council and the standing advisory committees.

- Maker of detailed rules, regulations, and orders (subject to the control of Parliament) by which the health service was to be controlled.
- Securer of parliamentary sanction for continued financing of the service, with added responsibilities of monitoring costs of the service, approving expenditure and reporting back to Parliament on matters of expenditure.
- Default and inquiry powers which gave sanction to decisions and requests.
- To acquire and own, on behalf of the government, land needed for the purposes of the Act.
- Responsible for all new legislation relating to the health services and many other matters relating to welfare and environmental health.

This vast degree of responsibility made the Minister the integral part of the NHS, without whom the various units could not function to provide a comprehensive and truly National Health Service.

The National Health Service Act 1946 relating to optical services

The ophthalmic services to be offered under this legislation were to be known as the supplementary ophthalmic services. The reason for this title was that the original ideal of the health service providing full eye care within the confines of the hospital eye service could not be achieved, and the Minister of Health established the Eye Services Committee whose function was to look at and report on:

1. The status, the scope of work and the designation of opticians in the final form of the national ophthalmic services as envisaged in the original National Health Service Act 1946.
2. The criteria to be applied when selecting opticians for appointment in the (temporary) supplementary eye services.

The Committee was composed of representatives of ophthalmologists, medical practitioners, and ophthalmic and dispensing opticians. The role of opticians in the proposed National Health Service was established on the basis of the Eye Services Committee report published in May 1947. As a result of the report, the Central Professional Committee for Opticians was established in November 1947, to consider all applications to work in the supplementary ophthalmic services. Any optician applying to work in the health services was required to give evidence of qualification and of adequate experience.

By the time the health service was operational in July of 1948, it became a duty of the newly formed Executive Councils to establish services in connection with the diagnosis and treatment of disease or defect of the eyes and the supply of optical appliances. To ensure an adequate specialist service the duties of the Executive Council in the field of ophthalmics were to be exercised on behalf of the Council by a committee called the Ophthalmic Services Committee.

Regulations were made to include provision for:

- The preparation and publication of lists of medical practitioners, of ophthalmic opticians and of dispensing opticians who undertook to provide supplementary ophthalmic services.
- Conferring the right of inclusion in the appropriate list on all having an eligible qualification.
- Conferring on any person the right to choose who should test his or her eyes and who should supply the prescribed appliance.
- The removal from the list of ophthalmic or dispensing opticians undertaking to provide supplementary ophthalmic services the name of any ophthalmic or dispensing optician who had never provided or who had ceased to provide such services.

The National Health Service Act 1946 also resulted in the establishment of an optical Whitley Committee, the purpose of which was to negotiate salaries for hospital opticians, fees for opticians working part time within the hospital eye service and fees for opticians working in the supplementary ophthalmic services.

Essentially, the original legislation set out to make provisions such that everyone was eligible for free eye examination and free spectacles within the supplementary ophthalmic services. Before this a relatively small percentage of people had been eligible for certain optical benefits by way of the additional benefit provisions of the National Health Insurance Acts.

Health Services and Public Health Act 1968

The Health Services and Public Health Act 1968 was intended:

> '*to amend the National Health Service Act 1946 and the National Health Services (Scotland) Act 1947, and make other amendments connected with the National Health Service; to make amendments connected with local authorities' services under the National Assistance Act 1948; to amend the law relating to notifiable diseases and food poisoning; to amend the Nurseries and Child Minders Regulation Act 1948; to amend the law relating to food and drugs; to enable assistance to be given to certain voluntary organisations; to enable the Minister of Health and the Secretary of State to purchase goods for supply to certain authorities; to make other amendments in the law relating to the public health; and for purposes connected with the matters aforesaid*'.

As can be seen, this was a wide-ranging piece of legislation.

Effect of the Health Services and Public Health Act 1968 on optical services

The effect of this legislation on the supplementary ophthalmic services was beneficial. The executive councils had their membership increased from 25 to 30, and for the first time one ophthalmic optician and one dispensing optician acted as representatives nominated from the local optical committee.

This legislation also put the ophthalmic services on a permanent footing; it became known as the general ophthalmic services and not the supplementary ophthalmic service. The old ophthalmic services committee, whose job (on behalf of the Executive Councils) had been to assess the qualifications of those wishing to offer ophthalmic services in areas where they were needed, could thus be dissolved. (This was included under the terms of the new Health Services and Public Health Act.) In addition, s.18(3) provided an amendment to the National Health Service Act 1946, allowing for the provisions of general ophthalmic services at health centres by ophthalmic medical practitioners, ophthalmic opticians, and dispensing opticians.

Finally, ophthalmic, and dispensing opticians were defined as follows.

1   'Ophthalmic optician' means a person listed in either of the registers, maintained under s.2 of the Opticians Act 1958, of ophthalmic opticians, or bodies corporate enrolled in the list, maintained under s.4 of the Opticians Act 1958, of such bodies carrying on business as ophthalmic opticians.
2   'Dispensing optician' means a person listed in the register, maintained under s.2 of the Opticians Act 1958, of dispensing opticians, or bodies corporate enrolled in the list, maintained under s.4 of the 1958 Opticians Act, of such bodies carrying on businesses as dispensing opticians.

National Health Service Reorganisation Act 1973

It was decided that, despite the amendments of the 1968 Act, and the fact that the NHS had certainly lived up to the four principles upon which it was based, there was a certain need for streamlining. Four objectives had to be met in the reorganisation:

1   The uniting of existing separate services, followed by their integration at local level.
2   The establishment of close links between the unified service and the public health and social services provided by local authorities.
3   The maximum responsibility for administering the service consistent with national plans and priorities should be placed on area health authorities. There should be strong local and professional participation and community involvement in the running of the services in any particular district.

4   The provision for effective central control over money spent on the service and to obtain maximum value.

It was decided that the NHS should be provided and financed by central government. This meant that a boundary had to be drawn between the types of services administered by the health authority and those administered by the local authority.

The National Health Service Reorganisation Act was eventually placed on the statute books in 1973. The new Act still placed the Minister at the head of the services but required also that the following should be provided:

- Hospital accommodation.
- Other accommodation for the purposes of any service provided under the National Health Service Acts.
- Medical, dental, nursing and ambulance services.
- Such other facilities for the care of expectant and nursing mothers and young children as are considered appropriate as part of the health service.
- Such facilities for the prevention of illness and for the care of persons suffering from illness as are considered appropriate as part of the health service. (These facilities replaced the arrangements made by the local health authorities under s.12 of the Health Services and Public Health Act 1968.)
- Such other services as are required for the diagnosis and treatment of illness.

In addition to the above provisions, there should be arrangements for regular and adequate checks of schoolchildren for both medical and dental health. A regular family planning service also was established.

The local administration set-up was now directly under the control of the Minister and in the form of:

- Regional health authorities.
- Area health authorities.
- Area health authorities (teaching) if any tuition was undertaken at the hospitals within the area.

In this administrative system the Minister could direct any of the authorities to carry out any function on his behalf related to the National Health Services Acts. The regional health authority could direct an area health authority within its own region to carry out any function relating to the National Health Service Acts, with the proviso that the Minister could counter such directive.

It became the task of the area health authorities to establish family practitioner committees (FPCs) to replace the executive councils and administer the provision of:

- General medical services.
- General dental services.
- General pharmaceutical services.
- General ophthalmic services.

The FPC comprised:

- Eleven members appointed by the area health authority.
- Four members appointed by the local authority (or jointly if two or more local authorities were entitled to appoint members).
- Eight members appointed by the local medical committee of whom one must be an ophthalmic medical practitioner.
- Three members appointed by the local dental committee.
- Two members appointed by the local pharmaceutical committee.
- One ophthalmic optician appointed by the local optical committee.
- One dispensing optician appointed by the local optical committee.

In addition to these, formal recognition was given to a committee where the Secretary of State was satisfied that it was formed for the regional health authority, as representative of any of the following:

- Medical practitioners of the region.
- Dental practitioners of the region.
- Nurses and midwives of the region.
- Registered pharmacists of the region.
- Registered ophthalmic and dispensing opticians of the region.
- Any group of representatives of other categories providing services.

Effect of the National Health Service Reorganisation Act 1973 on optometrists

As far as the ophthalmic services were concerned, this legislation had little effect. The local optical committee became a firmly established part of the area health authority and gave the optical profession a voice in the administrative system at local level. The only other change was simply one of name, with the executive council becoming the family practitioner committee without any alteration in the optical representation or duties.

National Health Service Act 1977

This Act was issued in order:

> '*to consolidate certain provisions relating to the health service for England and Wales; and to repeal certain enactments relating to the health service which have ceased to have any effect*'.

Part I of the Act dealt with services and administration at national and local levels. It set out the duties of the Secretary of State as regards health services. Also, under Part I the Secretary of State was required to establish councils termed community health councils, and it was a statutory duty that all parts of area health authorities be included within the district of a community health council. The composition of these councils was outlined in Sch. 7 of the Act, and the duties were:

1 To represent in the health service, the interests of the public in their district.
2 To perform other functions as laid down within the Schedule. These other functions were to include:
   (a) to visit and inspect premises controlled by the relevant area health authority:
   (b) to consider matters relating to the operation of the health service within their district and advise the area health authorities.
   (c) to prepare and publish reports on the operation of the health service within their district.

Part II of the National Health Service Act 1977 dealt specifically with general medical, general dental, general ophthalmic and pharmaceutical services. As far as the general ophthalmic services were concerned, the Act required that every area health authority arrange for medical practitioners with the prescribed qualifications and ophthalmic opticians to provide a service for the testing of sight and for suitably qualified ophthalmic and dispensing opticians to supply optical appliances.

Section 39 required that lists be drawn up of suitably qualified practitioners who would undertake to provide general ophthalmic services. Any person suitably qualified wishing to be included in the appropriate list should be so included. It also made provision for the general public to choose whomsoever they wished to test their eyes and whomsoever they wished to supply their appliance. A final note related to removal of the name of anyone included in the list who had never provided or who had ceased to provide such general ophthalmic services in the area.

Part III of the Act discussed other powers of the Secretary of State relating to the health service. Regulations relating to the changes for dental or optical appliances were laid down in s.78. that referred to para.2 of Sch.12 to this Act. The schedule gave details of the interpretation of the term 'current specified cost' as related to spectacle frames. It also listed details of exemptions from normal costs including children under 16 years of age or receiving full-time education in school. The information was related to the terms of service for ophthalmic opticians as laid down in SI 1974/287.

Part IV related to property and to finance for the health authorities.

Part V detailed the terms of service of a Health Service Commissioner for England and a Health Service Commissioner for Wales.

Part VI related to miscellaneous items not falling within these other categories.

Health Service Act 1980

The effect of this legislation was to replace the area health authorities with local district health authorities.

Health and Social Security Act 1984

This Act introduced the framework for a new set of terms of service that form the basis of those currently in use. It also withdrew the range of NHS frames and lenses that were available to eligible individuals and introduced in their place a voucher system for the provision of appliances.

Organisationally the status and constitution of the FPC's was amended.

For optics this Act was a major change to the way services had previously been supplied and should be considered as fundamental to the development of optical services.

Health and Medicines Act 1988

Another fundamental change to General Ophthalmic Services was introduced by this Act that withdrew the right of all individuals to a NHS sight test. The Act restricted eligibility categories for those entitled to a NHS sight test and moved the service towards privatisation.

Opticians Act 1989

This was a consolidation Act to pull together the legislation that had been enacted since the original Act of 1958. This Act will be discussed in detail in Chapter 6.

NHS and Community Care Act 1990

Following circulation of a discussion document from the NHS 'Working for Patients' FPCs were replaced by Family Health Service Authorities (FHSAs) upon implementation of the National Health Service and Community Care Act 1990. It was the responsibility of the FHSA to continue to administer the services previously provided by the FPC and to extend responsibility in relation to:

- Planning.
- Development and monitoring of primary health care services.

- Collaboration with other service agencies and local authority Social Services Departments.
- Implementation of the NHS white paper 'Caring for people' and the NHS and Community Care Act 1990.

The Act also changed the membership of the FHSA which in future would consist of:

- A Chairman appointed by the Secretary of State
- Four professional non-executive directors (one from each of the following service professions):
  - GP,
  - dentist.
  - pharmacist,
  - nursing.
- Five generalist non-executive directors appointed by the Regional Health Authority.
- General Manager of FHSA as an Executive Director.

Health Authorities Act 1995

This Act of Parliament abolished Regional Health Authorities, District Health Authorities and Family Health Service Authorities and replaced them with Health Authorities and Special Health Authorities. As far as optometry is concerned the effect of this was purely to change the title of the Authority controlling local arrangements.

National Health Service (Primary Care) Act 1997

An amendment was made to the Opticians Act 1989 via this 1997 Act. The effect of the amendment was minor but provided slightly more flexibility for referral.

Also, the National Health Service and Community Care Act 1990 was amended through this Act to specify that provision of Ophthalmic services by a person on the ophthalmic list fell within the context of a service under NHS contract.

Health Act 1999

Between December 1997 and October 1998, the Government published a series of papers on its proposals for the National Health Service in England, Scotland, and Wales. The documents were:

- Cm3807 The new NHS
- Cm3811 Designed to Care
- Cm3841 Putting Patients First
- HSC 1998/113 A First Class Service
- Partnership in Action (a discussion document)
- Quality Care and Clinical Excellence (a consultation document)
- Partnership in Improvement

Following on from these the Health Act 1999 received Royal assent in June 1999. It had far reaching consequences for the NHS and some specific amendments to regulations affecting optometry. The main purpose of the Act was to make changes to the way in which the National Health Service is run. GP fund holding was abolished and the Act paved the way for the establishment of new statutory bodies (Primary Care Trusts).

A new body was formed aimed at improving quality of care. The Commission for Health Improvement was established to monitor and help improve the quality of health care provided by the NHS.

The terms of the Act enable the Secretary of State to require general medical practitioners, general dental practitioners, optometrists, and pharmacists to hold approved indemnity cover. (This was an area that the GOC had already reviewed).

Changes were made in an attempt to tackle fraud in the NHS. A civil penalty was created that could be imposed where a person fails to pay an NHS charge or claims a payment to which he is not entitled towards the cost of an NHS charge or service. Further knowingly making false representations to evade or gain a reduction or remission of, or a payment relating to, NHS charges became a criminal offence. It also becomes possible for a body corporate or an individual practitioner to be disqualified from providing ophthalmic services locally or if considered appropriate nationally.

The final element of this legislation that could impact on optometry was a change to the format of making Orders in Council regarding regulation of health care professionals. This would allow for the GOC to put forward changes that would otherwise require Parliamentary debate and inclusion within an Act of Parliament for the Government to agree and introduce through Statutory Instrument.

Health and Social Care Act 2001

The Health and Social Care Act 2001 formally established care trusts as organisations which would commission and hold responsibility for local authority health-related functions and promote greater integration between health and local authority services.

The Act provided for primary care trusts (PCTs) and NHS trusts to be designated as care trusts in cases where they had local authority health-related functions delegated to them by agreement. Care trusts would commission and/or provide integrated services covering health, social services, and other health-related functions of a local authority. It was voluntary for local areas to establish care trusts. However, where joint working and services were failing, the Secretary of State for Health could direct local areas into partnership arrangements.

In relation to Optometry the listing arrangements were amended to include grounds on which a Health Authority may, or must, refuse to include a medical practitioner or an ophthalmic optician in a performer list and the information required on application and the details of an appeals process.

NHS Reform and Health Care Professions Act 2002

This Act reviewed and amended the NHS structure with Health Authorities in England becoming Strategic Health Authorities. In addition, a Commission for Patient and Public Involvement in Health was established, and this body would organise a local Patients' Forum for each NHS Trust and for each Primary Care Trust whose role would be to:

- monitor and review the range and operation of services provided by, or under arrangements made by, the trust for which it is established,
- obtain the views of patients and their carers about those matters and report on those views to the trust,
- provide advice, and make reports and recommendations, about matters relating to the range and operation of those services to the trust,
- make available to patients and their carers advice and information about those services,
- in prescribed circumstances, perform any prescribed function of the trust with respect to the provision of a service affording assistance to patients and their families and carers,
- carry out such other functions as may be prescribed.

A body corporate known as the Council for the Regulation of Health Care Professionals was also established with the general functions of:

- promoting the interests of patients and other members of the public in relation to the performance of their functions by the regulatory bodies mentioned (including the GOC) and by their committees and officers,
- promoting best practice in the performance of those functions,
- formulating principles relating to good professional self-regulation, and encouraging regulatory bodies to conform to them, and
- promoting co-operation between regulatory bodies and other bodies performing corresponding functions.

This had implications for optometry as the GOC was recognised as one of the regulatory bodies that would fall within the scope of action of the new Council.

Representative committees were to be recognised by PCT's. For optometry this meant that where a Primary Care Trust was satisfied that a committee formed for its area was representative of the ophthalmic opticians providing general ophthalmic services in the Primary Care Trust's area the Primary Care Trust may recognise that committee as the Local Optical Committee.

NHS Act 2006

The Act was essentially a consolidation of regulation on NHS structures and functions including developments in Primary Ophthalmic Services. Each PCT was required to provide or secure the provision, within its area, of a sight-testing service to meet the National requirements and such other primary ophthalmic services as may be prescribed. This enabled PCT's to commission services by way of General Ophthalmic Services contracts which would specify the services to be provided, the remuneration and any other relevant matters. The eligibility criteria for patient access to the sight-testing service were specified.

The legislation required that any performer of GOS eyecare services be listed by a PCT as an approved performer and the requirements for listing were specified. This led to the development of performer lists.

Local Optical Committees were included and under the legislation a PCT may recognise a committee formed for its area or one formed for its area and one or more other PCT areas providing the committee was representative of providers and performers involved in GOS in the area. The committees were able to delegate functions to subcommittees formed from its members and were also able to co-opt members who were not providers or performers if considered appropriate. The legislation also provided a mechanism for ensuring an annual review of funding by the PCT for administrative expenses including travel and subsistence for committee members. The LOC are obliged to provide to the PCT an annual review of its administrative expenditure to enable the PCT to fulfil its role.

Health Act 2006

This Act dealt with the introduction of a major no smoking policy in workplace settings and the signage to be required etc and formalised processes for counter fraud services both of which impact on optical services. More importantly for the optical professions it contained a section specific to General Ophthalmic Services and was the fore runner of the contractual changes that were subsequently made in 2008. The Act enabled a PCT to contract with any suitable person to provide services and could effectively provide primary services itself. Power was provided by the Act to enable provision to be made covering:

- the manner in which, and standards to which, GOS services were to be provided;
- the persons who perform services;
- the persons to whom services are to be provided;
- the variation of contract terms;
- rights of entry and inspection (including inspection of clinical records and other documents);
- the circumstances in which, and the manner in which, the contract may be terminated;
- enforcement;
- the adjudication of disputes.

An additional section included recognition of LOC's where a PCT in England was satisfied that the committee was representative of contractors and ophthalmic performers. A Primary Care Trust may be required by regulation as part of exercising its functions relating to primary ophthalmic services to consult any such committee it recognised under this section on such occasions and to such extent as may be prescribed.

Finally, from an optical perspective the Act also introduced clarification of actions following offences committed by officers or persons purporting to be officers of the body corporate. It also covered actions in partnerships and unincorporated associations (other than a partnership).

Health and Social Care Act 2008

This Act dissolved the Commission for Healthcare Audit and Inspection, the Commission for Social Care Inspection and the Mental Health Act Commission and the function of these bodies was taken over by a newly created Care Quality Commission.

The Act also established the office of the health professions adjudicator (OHPA), and this body's functions were to be discharged via fitness to practice panels. In the case of Optometry, the GOC were tasked with establishing membership of the panels according to the membership criteria in the Act, but the panels were to be independent of the GOC. Operational procedures for the panels were established by the Act. The OHPA was to be funded by the professional bodies involved and the OHPA would oversee and audit Fitness to Practice cases.

This Act introduced major changes to the monitoring and registration of Health and Social Care workers with the establishment of new bodies and new procedures across the whole healthcare sector.

Health Act 2009

This Act contained no specific changes to optical care and was aimed at implementing elements of the NHS Next Stage Review led by Lord Darzi. The Act covered aspects of the NHS constitution, annual quality accounts and enabled the Secretary of State to make monetary payment to patients in lieu of providing health care services to enable that patient to purchase their care directly from approved routes.

Health and Social Care Act 2012

The Act contains 12 Parts and 23 Schedules addressing a range of issues relating to Health and Social Care. It gives effect to the policies that were set out in the White Paper *Equity and Excellence: Liberating the NHS* which was published in July 2010. The main aims of the Act were to change how NHS care was commissioned through the greater involvement of clinicians and a new NHS Commissioning Board; to improve accountability and patient voice; to give NHS providers new freedoms to improve quality of care; and to establish a provider regulator to promote economic, efficient and effective provision and in addition take forward measures to reform public health services and health public bodies.

According to government documents *"The Health and Social Care Act 2012 puts clinicians at the centre of commissioning, frees up providers to innovate, empowers patients and gives a new focus to public health."*

It removed responsibility for the health of citizens from the Secretary of State for Health which the post had carried since the inception of the

NHS in 1948. It abolished primary care trusts (PCTs) and strategic health authorities (SHAs) in England and transferred "commissioning", or healthcare funds, from the abolished 152 PCTs to 211 GP led clinical commissioning groups. A new executive agency of the Department of Health, Public Health England, was established under the Act on 1 April 2013 and an independent NHS Board created to promote patient choice and to reduce NHS administration costs.

The Government emphasised that from the public's point of view nothing would change and access to NHS services based on need, not ability to pay, would continue.

The NHS Commissioning Board was the new body established to provide advice to CCGs on co-ordinating patient care. The Strategic Health Authorities (SHAs) that had existed to supervise PCTs were abolished, and the Care Quality Commission was tasked with ensuring that standards of care were maintained.

For optometry it provided opportunity to develop local commissioned services and to become involved in public health initiatives.

Health and Care Act 2022

The Health and Care Act, introduced into the House of Commons in July 2021 was intended to dismantle some of the structures established by the Health and Social Care Act 2012. Many of the proposals were intended to reinforce the ambitions of the NHS Long Term Plan. Implementation was delayed until July 2022.

The Act unpicks elements of the 2012 Act and the changes were aimed at supporting NHS organisations to collaborate to improve care and manage resources meaning the abolition of clinical commissioning groups (CCGs) and new area-based agencies being established. The Act puts "Integrated Care Systems" (ICS) on a statutory footing and merges NHS England and NHS Improvement.

An Integrated Care Board (ICB) and an integrated care partnership are established in every part of England. Each Board would be required to have, as a minimum:

- Four executives — the chief executive and finance, nursing, and medical directors.
- Three independent non-executives: a chair and at least two others. They "will normally not hold positions or offices in other health and care organisations within the ICS footprint".
- Three "partner members": one from an NHS trust/foundation trust in the patch, one from general practice, and one from a local authority.

The Act also includes provisions which would give the Secretary of State for Health and Social Care more power to direct NHS agencies, including NHS England and NHS Improvement, and over local service reconfigurations.

There is a potential for this to impact on Optometry through the commissioning of services by the newly created ICS but this remains to be seen as the system settles.

A brief note on Regional variation of NHS optometry services in the UK

The foregoing section has dealt with legislation passed by Parliament in London, and although there was until recently little variation in the regions these regulations apply specifically to England. During the development of the National Health Service as mentioned in the introduction there have been, for either environmental or political reasons, separate sets of regulations to cover Scotland, Wales, and Northern Ireland. As political devolution progressed in the UK and health care was provided as a devolved function the regulations covering these three Regions and the NHS has become different from the England based regulation and different from each other.

Aspects of NHS care and particularly supplementary services have expanded in all 3 Regions of the UK whilst remaining relatively static and disjointed in England. Core GOS sight testing services however are currently still reasonably consistent across all jurisdictions. Although the text is based on the position in England a very brief review of the NHS service provision in each of the other three UK Regions is provided below.

Scotland

Although separate legislation has existed for the NHS in Scotland for some time, for the most part the general ophthalmic services provided had been consistent with those in England, Northern Ireland, and Wales. The original legislative framework for the NHS in Scotland was set out in the National Health Service (Scotland) Act 1978.

On 1st April 2006, the NHS (General Ophthalmic Services) (Scotland) Regulations SI 2006/135 were established. This provided the fundamental basis for the provision of NHS primary services for eye care in Scotland in terms of who would perform and content etc. Under the regulation everyone in Scotland became eligible for a fully funded comprehensive NHS primary eye examination and not only exempted groups as elsewhere. The traditional NHS "sight test" previously available and consistent with other UK Regions was replaced by a comprehensive eye examination appropriate to the patient's needs. Under this system an initial eye examination could be carried out (primary eye examination) and where necessary a second eye examination (supplementary eye examination) with separate fees claimable. The system differs from other Regions in that it is available to all patients and not just those in exempt groups

Significant differences exist also in the administrative structure and in the provision of services for remote areas.

Under the devolved executive there are 14 Health Boards representing different areas and a single national Public Health Agency. When established it was envisaged that four main measures would be taken to pull together the work of primary care, acute services, and health improvement the different component parts of the local NHS system. These four principal measures are:

- Making all parts of the local NHS system accountable through the new NHS Board
- Introduction of a single Local Health Plan to ensure a more consistent and cohesive approach to planning

- A new performance and accountability framework
- Revised financial arrangements

In Scotland the 14 geographically based NHS Boards are responsible for both planning and delivering NHS services. There are also 14 Area Optometric Committees whose role is to provide professional and clinical advice to Health Boards and the Scottish Government. The NHS in Scotland provides universal access to a primary eye care service as part of General Ophthalmic Services (GOS) Scotland.

The GOS primary eye examination (PEE), supplementary eye examination (SEE) and enhanced supplementary eye examination (ESEE) are available nationally. This structure enables optometry to provide patients with routine, chronic or emergency eye conditions with the care and support they need and then to appropriately triage as clinically necessary. Transferring care out of hospitals and into the community has enabled optometrists to manage a greater range of eye conditions, as well as 'freeing up' GP appointments and reducing the pressure on the hospital eye service. Optometrists can also refer patients directly to hospital eye services where they deem necessary. Advisory committees will still play an important role in the function of the Boards and an optometric adviser has been appointed to the Scottish Executive.

There are enhanced services commissioned and funded at a local level, which means that there is some geographical variation. A review of Eye Care Services was undertaken in 2017 and a report (Community eye-care services: review 2017) published on the successful developments and future visions for eyecare in Scotland.

Optometrists in Scotland must be listed as performers in Scotland to perform services and are limited to performing a maximum of 20 eye examinations per day. The GOS contract in Scotland has a tiered fee structure. There is funding to support the training of independent prescribing (IP) optometrists, and the issuing of NHS prescribing pads to optometrists in 2013 ensured that the Scottish optometrist can manage ocular conditions within primary care at no cost to the patient.

The devolution of power to Scotland has impacted on the way eyecare services are provided expanding scope significantly and the latest review is likely to see further development in the future and it is therefore important to confirm the NHS situation if looking to practice in Scotland.

Northern Ireland

As with Scotland, the major differences between the ophthalmic services of Northern Ireland and those of England lie in the administrative structure, headed by the Northern Ireland Department of Health and Social Services. The Health and Social Care Board (HSCB) has contracts with over 250 ophthalmic practices across the region to provide general ophthalmic services for Health Service patients. The HSCB also plans and develops a range of special enhanced services to help manage increasing demands for eye health services (Curran 2017).

The Northern Ireland Eyecare Network is the successor to the Developing Eyecare Partnerships (DEP) Project, which was implemented in 2012 to improve how eyecare services were commissioned and delivered in Northern Ireland (NIEN 2021). The Eyecare Network's aim is "to reduce preventable sight loss by ensuring regionally integrated planning, commissioning, delivery, performance management, and funding of eyecare in Northern Ireland." The Northern Ireland Eyecare Network was formally constituted in January 2021 and is hosted by the Health and Social Care Board with leadership from:

- Health and Social Care Board;
- Public Health Agency;
- Clinicians from the two provider Trusts for Eyecare Services — Belfast Health and Social Care Trust and Western Health and Social Care Trust;
- RNIB

Local Enhanced eye care is provided by optometrists and all optometrists practicing in Northern Ireland are required to be listed as performers in Northern Ireland.

Wales

The National Assembly for Wales (Transfer of Functions) Order 1999 SI 1999/672 has moved many of the functions of the Secretary of State in relation to the NHS to the National Assembly for Wales.

Wales has established Local Health Groups (equivalent to primary Care Groups/Trusts in England) to act as the providers of primary care.

Recognising the increasing gap between the demand for, and capacity to provide, specialist hospital eye care services, Wales took the decision to utilise optometrists for non-GOS services and the Wales Eye Care Initiative was launched in May 2002 bringing together the Primary Eye Care Acute Referral Scheme (PEARS) and an enhanced examination for groups at risk of developing eye disease, including:

- people with sight in only one eye
- people with a hearing impairment
- people who suffer from retinitis pigmentosa
- people whose family origins are Black African, Black Caribbean, Indian, Pakistani, and Bangladeshi.

The PEARS scheme initially developed as a pilot by optometric practices in the Vale of Glamorgan, enabled optometrists to become the first point of contact for acute eye conditions in primary care, allowing optometrists to manage a range of non sight-threatening conditions and alleviate pressures on general practitioners. Referral routes to the hospital eye service (HES) were simultaneously revised, with direct referral from optometrist to HES becoming standard across Wales.

The routine dilation of patients, use of a binocular indirect retinal examination, threshold visual field testing and Goldmann tonometry, formed the basis of the enhanced provision for at-risk groups, with an emphasis on early detection of eye disease and improved outcomes for patients, with services being provided free of charge through the NHS.

Eye care services continued to develop with the introduction of the Low Vision Service Wales in 2003.

Eye health services have further evolved and developed into the Wales Eye Care Services (WECS) encompassing Eye Health Examination Wales (EHEW), Low Vision Service Wales (LVSW) and Diabetic Eye Screening Wales (DESW).

Eye Health Examination Wales comprises three service elements:

Band 1 encompassing the initial services provided under WECS as described above.

Band 2 allowing for referral refinement of a number of conditions following a GOS or private examination e.g., glaucoma repeat measurements, dilated cataract refinement and counselling.

Band 3 allowing optometrists to follow-up patients after initial acute presentations and facilitate the HES to discharge patients for postoperative cataract assessment in primary care.

A manual of services has been produced and updated (EHEW manual 2018) by NHS Wales for those involved in primary eye health care covering aspects of Service Information, Service Protocols, Service Guidance and Clinical Guidance. The manual deals with protocols for eyecare provision beyond the basic GOS primary care sight test.

Chapter 2

The NHS General Ophthalmic Services Contract England

For most optometrists in the UK much of their time will be spent working with patients who are eligible for General Ophthalmic Services (GOS) sight tests under the National Health Service (NHS). Few optometry practices currently survive by seeing private patients exclusively although this may change in the future if optometry follows the route of dentistry privatisation in the UK.

Figures for the year to April 2014 (the latest reliable data) indicated that the percentage split of NHS to private examinations was 71/29 (*Optics at a Glance* FODO). The graph below (Fig 1) shows the change in the number of NHS sight tests as a percentage of the total number of sight tests performed from estimates published in Optics at a Glance with a starting point in April 1989–March 1990 of 41%. This figure of 41% was at a time of changes to the eligibility criteria for NHS testing introduced by the Health and Medicines Act 1988 and at a time when the total number of sight tests had fallen significantly. The impact of government changes is again shown in the 1998-1999 figures when the announcement a year ahead of implementation that over 60-year-olds would be eligible for NHS sight tests from April 1999 resulted in a drop in overall testing and a fall in the percentage of NHS tests performed with a bounce back over the following year. From 2001-2002 there has been a small increase

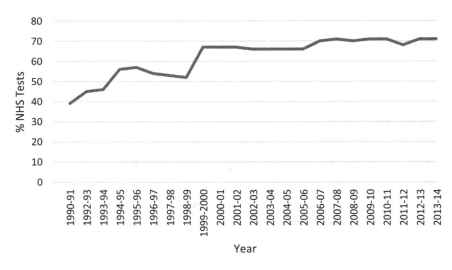

Figure 1:   NHS sight tests as a percentage of the total number of sight tests performed in the UK by year

in the percentage of NHS tests although this was stable at around 70% of the total number of tests performed for the last 7 years of data available.

Other factors that should be considered when reviewing the data are that until 2007 the figures for Northern Ireland were not included in the data and from 2006 a NHS sight test in Scotland was available to all. Although the changes in Scotland resulted in a significant rise of 64% in the numbers of NHS sight tests in that Region, this, and the inclusion of figures for Northern Ireland did not significantly impact the total, providing a rise in NHS activity of some 8% at a time when the rise in total numbers of sight tests NHS and private across the UK was approximately 5%.

This chapter is based on the requirements to provide GOS sight tests in England and as mentioned in Chapter 1 there are variations across the Regions in the UK to some elements particularly the administrative structure. In England a provider must obtain a contract with NHS England for the area in which they wish to use appropriate fixed premises (Mandatory Services Contract) or offer domiciliary services (Additional Services Contract). A contractor may choose to apply for either a mandatory services contract or an additional services contract or both. Similar arrangements are in place in the other 3 regions of the UK. A Contractor does not need to be a registered health professional to receive a contract and may own multiple practices. However, any contractor in England may only use a registered performer to perform sight testing and the performer must appear on the NHS England performer list (a performer appearing on lists in Scotland, Wales or Northern Ireland would require to be listed also in England to perform services in England). There are similar arrangements in place for Scotland, Northern Ireland, and Wales.

What is the Contract?

Essentially the contract provides for NHS England to make payments to a listed contractor for the delivery of primary ophthalmic services provided within the scope of the NHS. Primary ophthalmic services in this context relate only to the testing of sight. In return for such payments the contractor agrees to comply with the conditions as set out in the National Health Service, England General Ophthalmic Services Contracts Regulations 2008 (SI 2008 No 1185) and subsequent amendments. As a result, patients are provided with local ophthalmic services to a recognised standard and the hospital eye service is not inundated with patients seeking sight testing.

Originally GOS services were provided via a contract with an individual Primary Care Trust (PCT), but this changed following the formation of the National Health Service Commissioning Board in 2013. The Board is a statutory body established by the National Health Service Act 2006. It is the duty of the Board to exercise its powers to secure the provision throughout England of mandatory primary ophthalmic services. The Board became known as NHS England in April 2013. By virtue of a property transfer scheme made under s.300 of the Health and Social Care Act 2012, all general ophthalmic services contracts entered into before 1st April 2013 transferred to the Board on that date.

The requirements of the contract refer to both clinical and non-clinical aspects of a practice. Contracts may be for solely Mandatory, solely Additional or both services. These are discussed below.

Parties to the contract

As mentioned above anyone can apply for a contract to provide GOS sight testing whether a registered practitioner or not. the application however must specify:

- the names of the parties applying for the contract;
- the type of contract applied for i.e., whether the contract is for mandatory services or for additional services or for both; in the case of a partnership —
- whether or not it is a limited partnership, and
- the names of the partners and, in the case of a limited partnership, their status as a general or limited partner; and
- in the case of each party, the postal address to which official correspondence and notices should be sent.

The contractor must not use any name for the business that is subject to a disqualification and must not use any protected title or imply registration with the regulatory body when not registered.

Premises for providing GOS sight testing services

An application for a contract may include any number of premises for listing in which sight testing services are provided however all premises and the equipment in each location must be:

- suitable to enable delivery of sight testing
- sufficient to meet reasonable needs of patients
- able to offer suitable and sufficient waiting room accommodation for patients
- able to provide any other facilities necessary to perform the service

A contractor is approved only to provide general ophthalmic services at an address that is included in his/her entry in the ophthalmic list or, if an additional contract is held, at the residential address of a patient eligible for a domiciliary visit or at certain specified day centres or residential homes. If services are to be provided at another location a separate application must be made for the new address to be included in the ophthalmic list.

As mentioned above "Suitable and sufficient" waiting and consulting room accommodation and suitable equipment for provision of GOS must be provided. No criteria are available to define "suitable and sufficient" and this will be determined initially by NHS England before a contract is issued and then at any point as part of contract monitoring. The terms of the contract require the contractor to admit an authorised officer of NHS England who has made a written request to inspect accommodation or equipment at all reasonable times.

Performers

A contractor may employ or engage an ophthalmic practitioner to perform sight testing services under GOS but must ensure that the performer is included in an appropriate ophthalmic performer list and is registered with the appropriate regulatory body and not under suspension and has suitable references. The contractor has a responsibility to ensure that the performer is suitably qualified and competent to perform the services. Should the performer be working under "conditions" issued either by the regulatory body or by the listing authority then the contractor must ensure that these conditions are being met. Performers should notify any employers of conditions should they be imposed. Performers must be listed in the Region in which they test sight i.e., to sight test under GOS in England the performer must appear on the list for England.

To be accepted on to a list a performer must be registered with the General Optical Council and have successfully completed the relevant application process. In England the administrative process is undertaken by Primary Care Services England and once completed the application requires NHS England approval. Guidance on the application process for England can be found at https://indd.adobe.com/view/4139f1e8-ecbb-4457-9b30-f398ea7e8cb8.

To work as an optometrist in Northern Ireland and provide General Ophthalmic Services in a contractor practice, an applicant will need to formally apply to the Health and Social Care Board in order to be eligible to provide GOS.

To work as an optometrist in Scotland, an applicant will need to obtain a General Ophthalmic Services contract in Scotland via a Health Service Board. This requires completion of a GOS Competency Training Assessment which is a practical assessment carried out on a live patient.

To work as an optometrist in Wales providing General Ophthalmic Services an applicant must complete the OPL1 application form to be included in the ophthalmic list and submit it to NHS Wales Shared Services Partnership.

Testing of sight

Under the contract regulations 2008 a contractor who is listed as providing GOS sight testing is required to arrange for the testing of sight of any eligible patient where a test is considered clinically necessary. The testing of sight should be to determine whether the patient needs to wear or use an optical appliance and should comply with the duties imposed by the Opticians Act 1989. The contractor is responsible for ensuring in addition to patient eligibility that a sight test is necessary. No patient is "automatically entitled" to a GOS sight test and both the eligibility and "necessary" criteria must be met.

Having completed a GOS sight test the contractor is responsible for ensuring that the patient is given a copy of the outcome of the sight-test and this prescription may be taken and used elsewhere should the patient make that choice. It is a breach of the Opticians Act and therefore the GOS contract to either require a patient to agree to purchasing a product in advance as a condition of performing the sight test should one be necessary or to refuse to issue a prescription should the patient wish to purchase an appliance elsewhere.

Any prescription issued following the sight test must be in the form recommended in Appendix A to the BS 2738 Part 3 :2004 and must comply with any requirements issued by the Secretary of State. Although the NHS use a standard form (GOS2) for issue to a patient with details of the findings of the sight test the regulations do not specify that the NHS form must be used. Since the introduction of electronic submission of forms, it has become more likely that a contractor will use their own design format for the prescription. If using a different format however the details included in any prescription issued must comply with the requirements of the Opticians Act 1989 and SI 1989/1230.

According to The Sight Testing (Examination and Prescription) (No 2) Regulations 1989 (SI 1989/1230) any prescription provided following a sight test complying with the Opticians Act must include:

1. Details of the lenses prescribed
2. Date of testing of sight
3. Name and address of the patient and if under 16 their date of birth
4. Name of the optometrist who carried out the testing of sight and details including the address of the practice where the sight test took place
5. A statement of no change if there is no prescription change or an insignificant prescription change

Records

As part of the GOS contract requirements a contractor agrees to keep a proper record concerning each patient to whom GOS are provided. This must provide a full, accurate and contemporaneous record giving appropriate details of the testing of sight. The record may be in hard copy or electronic format.

It is also a requirement that all such records are maintained for a minimum period of seven years (although not required by the contract this period may (and should) be extended for certain patient categories). To enable audit and monitoring of the contract, if required, the contractor must produce the record for any authorised officer representing NHS England within a specified period that will not be less than 14 days. Regular audits are undertaken on behalf of NHS England, and it is therefore crucial that records are contemporaneous, accurate, well maintained and meet the requirements of the contract.

The topics of records and record keeping are covered in greater detail in Chapter 12.

Informing and referral

The GOS contract deals with information and referral requirements where on examination:

- a patient shows signs of injury, disease, or abnormality in the eye or elsewhere which may require medical treatment, or
- a satisfactory standard of vision is not achieved even when using corrective lenses.

These requirements are changing rapidly with the development of supplementary contracted services but, in the absence of any alternative agreed pathway, when an optometrist feels that further investigation/management is required a referral should be made to the patient's GP. If the optometrist feels it more appropriate for them to monitor the situation in their practice, then the patients GP should be informed of this. In addition, if considered appropriate, and with the consent of the patient a performer may refer the patient to an ophthalmic hospital or an ophthalmic department of a hospital and notify the GP practice that this has been done although care must be taken that this remains within locally accepted pathways. A considerable number of schemes have been established to provide triaging/refining of referrals in eye care and it is important to be aware of the systems available in any area where services are to be performed.

A referral form (GOS 18) produced by the NHS is available for patient referrals but alternatively many practices have their own systems for producing a letter. When making a referral the optometrist is required to provide the patient with a written statement of the details of the referral and often this takes the form of a copy of the referral letter. Referral is covered in more detail in Chapter 12. The NHS regulations run in parallel with the GOC regulations (see Chapter 7) but unlike the GOC rules are only relevant to patients seen within the GOS.

Application by a patient for GOS mandatory services

The GOS contract enables a contractor to provide mandatory services to any eligible person where a sight test is considered necessary. In the case of a child a request for services may be made on their behalf by:

- either parent;
- a person duly authorised by a local authority to whose care the child has been committed under the Children Act 1989(a); or
- a person duly authorised by a voluntary organisation which is accommodating the child under the provisions of the Children Act 1989.

In the case of an adult who is incapable of making an application or authorising an application to be made on their behalf the request may be made by:

- a relative or
- the primary carer of the person.

It is the responsibility of the contractor to be satisfied that the person is eligible for the service by asking for satisfactory evidence of eligibility unless, in cases other than where the patient is a person of limited resources, satisfactory evidence of eligibility is already available. This may be for example by referring to previous records or by measuring the power of the lenses of the person's existing optical appliance if a complex prescription.

If a patient has been asked for, but not produced, evidence and there is no other satisfactory evidence of eligibility this fact should be recorded on the patient's GOS sight test form. This does not prevent the contractor from providing the service but puts the onus on proving eligibility onto the patient — there is a "fine" that the NHS can impose for false declaration of eligibility and the patient should be warned of this.

As part of the check for eligibility it is the responsibility of the contractor prior to testing to ensure that the details of the patient and the approximate date of the last sight test (whether under GOS or privately and whether in the UK or overseas) is correctly recorded on the appropriate GOS 1 sight test form by the patient or on their behalf.

It is a breach of the GOS contract to advise an eligible person that mandatory services are not available or to mislead the patient about the availability, quality and extent of the services provided under the contract with a view to obtaining the agreement of a patient to undergo services privately.

Are there circumstances under which GOS may be refused?

Services under the contract may be refused to an eligible person where a contractor has reasonable grounds to refuse, and the grounds should be identified on the patient record. Suitable reasons may be for example where a patient is too intoxicated to undertake testing or is violent or abusive to staff or other patients. Where refusal occurs however those grounds cannot relate to a person's:

- race, gender, social class, age, religion, sexual orientation, appearance, disability or medical or ophthalmic condition; or
- a decision or intended decision to accept or refuse private services in respect of themselves or a family member.

Entitlement v Eligibility

Patients in specific groups who are eligible for a GOS sight test are entitled to have the sight test funded by the NHS. The entitlement therefore is to NHS funding where appropriate and not an entitlement to a GOS sight test and this generates confusion for both patient and contractor. The final decision on eligibility lies with a contractor who according to the NHS contract must satisfy themselves that in addition to falling within one of the entitlement groups a sight test is clinically necessary and appropriate. Patients entitled to NHS funding for example would not normally be eligible for a sight test at an interval of less than 2 years. The groups covered by the entitlement to a NHS funded sight test are defined within Statutory Instrument 1986/975 and subsequent amendments as persons who:

- are under 16 years of age
- under the age of 19 years and receiving qualifying full-time education — the cut-off point for educational eligibility is the end of the summer term but for those changing educational activities (e.g., going on to higher education) it has been agreed as the September following the end of the normal summer term. This means that students continuing in education state their last school as their educational establishment until they confirm their place for the next academic year.
- are 60 years of age or over
- are registered as partially sighted or blind
- have been diagnosed with diabetes or glaucoma — this category includes:
  - o patients who previously have suffered from diabetes, but the condition is considered to be treated
  - o patients with high intraocular pressure who have been advised by their ophthalmologist that they are at risk of glaucoma even though it is not currently present.
- are 40 years of age or over and their mother, father, a sibling, or child has been diagnosed with glaucoma
- are a prisoner on leave from prison
- are eligible for an NHS complex lens voucher
- are or are the partner of someone — including civil partner — or are under 20 years of age and the dependant of someone receiving:
  - Income Support
  - Income-related Employment and Support Allowance
  - Income-based Jobseeker's Allowance
  - Pension Credit Guarantee Credit
  - Universal Credit and meet the criteria
  - are entitled to or named on:
  - a valid NHS tax credit exemption certificate
  - a valid NHS certificate for full help with health costs (HC2)

People named on an NHS certificate for partial help with health costs (HC3) may also be entitled to funding towards the cost of a private sight test.

Changes to a contract and notifications to NHS England

Contractors have a duty to keep up to date with changes in GOS arrangements and normally these will be sent to the registered address by NHS England. As contractors and performers are required to notify NHS England of all changes in address this should not be a problem. However, should a contractor or performer fail to keep their details up to date and changes are distributed but not received, the individual will be considered at fault if he/she fails to comply. It is essential therefore for a contractor to ensure all address changes be notified. Ignorance through non-receipt due to failure to notify a change of address is not a defence.

The contractor is required to notify NHS England as soon as reasonably practicable, of any serious incident that affects or is likely to affect the Contractor's performance of its obligations under the Contract. This may be due to premises issues such as a flood or fire requiring the normal services to be withdrawn for a period or preventing the contractor meeting the sufficient and suitability criteria or may be due to equipment failure that would prevent a sight test being completed (e.g., no visual field equipment available for a period of time).

Where circumstances arise that would give rise to the right to terminate the contract by NHS England or where the information relating to the contractor that NHS England publish change then NHS England should be notified. This may relate to times that the GOS service is available or to changes in performers listed.

Additional requirements for a corporate body

Where the Contractor is a corporate body, the contractor should notify NHS England when:

- it passes a resolution, or a court of competent jurisdiction makes an order that the Contractor be wound up;

- circumstances arise that might entitle a creditor or a court to appoint a receiver, administrator, or administrative receiver for the Contractor;
- circumstances arise which would enable a court to make a winding up order in respect of the Contractor;
- the Contractor is unable to pay its debts within the meaning of section 123 of the Insolvency Act 1986; or
- a new director, chief executive or secretary of the corporate body is appointed — this notification should confirm that any new director etc meets the required conditions.

Additional requirements for a partnership

In the case of a partnership the Contractor should notify NHS England when:

- a partner leaves or informs the partners of an intention to leave the partnership — the notification should include the date on which the partner left or the proposed leaving date
- a new partner joins or proposes to join the partnership — the notification should
  - o state the date that the new partner joined, or it is proposed will join the partnership;
  - o state whether the new partner is an ophthalmic practitioner;
  - o confirm that the new partner meets the required conditions of a partner and include an appropriate application form
  - o state whether the new partner is or is to be a general or limited partner.

Notices to be displayed

A contractor must ensure that a notice supplied or approved by NHS England is displayed prominently in a patient area indicating the services available under the GOS contract. The notice should include details of eligibility and any charges relevant to GOS services.

A further notice should be displayed providing information on the complaints procedure within the practice and providing the name and title of the person nominated by the contractor to deal with complaints.

Details of business ownership should be displayed in an area that is prominent and visible to patients. Frequently the notice is placed in the main window of the practice or at the reception desk.

A Health and Safety poster should be displayed where it can be seen by any member of the practice team. The notice should meet standard format requirements and indicate the name of the person responsible for health and safety issues at the practice.

Insurance details providing information about the insurance cover for the practice should be displayed appropriately.

Complaints

The standard NHS provided poster indicating GOS eligibility criteria also includes details of the NHS complaints process. If this poster is not used, then details of the contact details for making a complaint should be displayed where they are clearly visible to a patient. The GOS contract requires a NHS compliant complaints procedure to be in place. Details of the procedure are found in the Local Authority Social Services and National Health Service Complaints [England] Regulations (2009). The same procedure should cover locally commissioned NHS services.

Template documentation and advice to assist contractors with complying with the requirements have been produced by the NHS (see https://www.england.nhs.uk › uploads › 2016/07/nhse-complaints-policy-june-2017.pdf) and the Optical Confederation now available on the FODO website.

Under the terms of the GOS contract each contractor must:

- take responsibility for the arrangements for dealing with complaints and designate a complaints manager
- inform the public of the arrangements and this may be via the GOS notice as mentioned above
- seek to resolve complaints in good faith and treat complainants appropriately — it is important to remember that GOS complaints relate to sight testing only there are separate routes available for complaints relating to dispensing appliances.

A complaint may be made up to twelve months after the incident in question and when received a contractor must:

- acknowledge receipt of the complaint within three working days
- offer to discuss the complaint with the complainant. Whether or not a meeting with the complainant takes place, the complainant must be informed about how the complaint is to be dealt with and how long it is expected take
- try to resolve the complaint within six months
- keep a record of all the complaints received
- submit details of all GOS complaints annually to NHS England.

Telephone services

With changes in circumstances and technology enabling for example telephone triaging the contractor should not use telephone services that relate to the GOS contract services unless provided free to the caller.

Safety of the public

To ensure consistency and standards of safety the contractor has responsibility for ensuring a safe environment, making appropriate arrangements for infection control and decontamination, and putting in place any relevant requirements of the Medicines and Healthcare products Regulatory Agency (MHRA) or the Health and Safety Executive.

As part of this responsibility the contractor must establish and operate arrangements to ensure that any ophthalmic practitioner who performs services under the contract and any other person employed by the contractor to perform or assist in the performance of services under the contract:

- Are aware of and use effective measures of infection control
- satisfy all legal requirements relating to health and safety in the workplace; and

- adhere to any requirements of or recommendations by the MHRA
- follows required waste disposal processes.

Withdrawing from the contract

A contractor wishing to withdraw from the list needs to give written notice to NHS England and normally will be withdrawn from the list after 3 months providing there are no outstanding issues with the contract. It may be possible in some circumstances to reduce this notice period by mutual agreement between the contractor and NHS England. In the case of a contractor dying or otherwise ceasing to be an Ophthalmic Medical Practitioner or Optometrist the name will be removed from the list 6 months after services cease to be provided.

The development of e-GOS

Since its inception GOS has been based around paper forms and documentation — however in October 2020 following a series of trials a computer-based system e-GOS went live with the intention of all practices being on the system by the end of 2021. This was always an ambitious target as not all practices were computerised! By January 2022 however most contractors were using the system although there were significant early issues resulting in mixed electronic and paperwork systems operating. The major benefits of an electronic system in addition to the reduced use of paper are the ability to analyse data in real time and the ability to review more accurately to determine fraudulent claiming.

The system is web-based and works on PC, mobile, tablet, iPad, and android, etc. However, you need a touch screen device that can be used to collect the required patient and contractor signatures.

Users will log in to the secure area of the PCSE website with their individual username and password, select the appropriate GOS form and complete the necessary details. The information for completing the online GOS forms is the same as is currently required for the paper forms, but the electronic system will automatically validate each entry. Any missing information, errors or incomplete mandatory fields will be flagged up before a form can be submitted, significantly reducing the likelihood of claims being rejected and improving the accuracy of payments.

Regulations have been changed to allow GOS forms to be signed electronically by the patient, optometrist, and contractor.

If a patient brings in a GOS3 from a practice that is using the new e-payment services, the voucher will appear different to previous vouchers and includes a unique reference number and authorisation code. If a practice is using PCSE Online or eGOS, then a search can be made online for a new style GOS3 using the reference number and authorisation code. The GOS 3 claim process can then be continued on PCSE Online or eGOS.

Where a practice is not using PCSE Online or eGOS as before the remainder of the GOS3 should be completed by hand and submitted with any other paper GOS3 forms as normal, with the appropriate batch header attached. It is acceptable for the GOS3 to be printed in black and white or full colour.

Contract for additional services (domiciliary)

A contractor applying for an Additional services contract is required to meet all the relevant standards in the mandatory contract — obviously some such as premises will not be applicable. In addition, there are several variations in the way that the contract operates.

Eligibility for domiciliary visits

In addition to the eligibility criteria for GOS listed for the mandatory contract to be eligible for domiciliary care the patient also must be unable to leave home unaccompanied. When claiming for a domiciliary visit the contractor must specify the clinical condition that enables the patient to meet this requirement.

Notification of visit Locations

As there are no fixed premises an additional services contractor is required to notify to NHS England in advance of attendance for appointments the locations to be visited and in the case of residential care homes the numbers of patients to be seen. This may well change over time as the system for post payment verification develops.

Who can request a visit?

Often a patient to be seen under additional services lacks capacity and care must be taken over who is arranging the visit. Normally it would be expected that a visit is requested by a relative or carer with power of attorney so that any decisions made following the visit are taken by the correct person with legal responsibility. It is not considered reasonable for a care home (or contractor) to arrange "block" attendance to perform sight tests and each patient should be treated as an individual event and meet the requirements.

Equivalence for additional services

It is expected from the contract that the level of care and the content of a sight test will be independent of the location at which it is performed. Therefore, although it may be different to meet the different circumstances it will be expected that adequate equipment is available to provide a clinically robust eyesight test wherever the location.

Performer listing

To perform GOS a registered optometrist must apply for separate listing in the area in which the services are to be supplied (i.e., England, Northern Ireland, Scotland, or Wales). All performers once listed are required to give an undertaking to comply with the regulations laid down for NHS contractors in addition to complying with any general regulation that applies to optometrists. Although it is the responsibility of the contractor to ensure compliance with the contract requirements if a performer is shown to have failed to meet any of the requirements, then action may be taken against the performer as an individual. It is therefore essential that all performers are aware of the full contract requirements.

The following information normally is recorded in the performer list:

- the ophthalmic practitioner's full name;
- the ophthalmic practitioner's professional registration number;
- confirmation of whether the ophthalmic practitioner is a contractor under a general ophthalmic services contract;
- if the ophthalmic practitioner is an ophthalmic medical practitioner, confirmation of that fact and the date of the practitioner's approval as an ophthalmic medical practitioner under regulation 43 or 44; and
- the date that the ophthalmic practitioner was first included in one of the following lists—
  o the ophthalmic performers list,
  o an ophthalmic performers list kept by a Primary Care Trust prior to the transfer date, or
  o an ophthalmic list or ophthalmic supplementary list, specifying which list.

NHS action for failure to comply with requirements

The effect of applying for and being included in the ophthalmic list as a contractor or as a performer is to accept the relevant terms of the NHS contract. Failure to comply with the terms would be considered as a breach of the contract. A number of actions are open to NHS England where a breach may have occurred, and action will depend on the severity and nature of the breach.

In the past investigations into for example alleged fraud have detected examples of submission of forms for non-existent patients or falsely claiming for domiciliary visits. Such cases in addition to being considered a breach of contract may be taken forward by NHS England to the Courts as a criminal offence.

In clinical cases involving performers (such as failure to complete a satisfactory examination) it is possible for NHS England to establish a local process of investigation and if considered appropriate establish a panel review. The NHS processes involve Performance Advisory Groups (PAG), and Performer List Disciplinary Panels (PLDP) and these are discussed in detail in Chapter 5. In some cases, the NHS process may be followed by full Tribunal Hearings.

Chapter 3

The GOS Memorandum of Understanding for Optometry

In November 1997 the Department of Health (DoH) issued FPN 713 as part of the introduction of revised General Ophthalmic Services (GOS) forms and in an attempt to offer clearer guidance on interpretation of GOS provision. As part of that advice section 22 of the Annex to the document states:

"In the Department's view adult patients with refractive errors, who do not have any underlying disease or risk of disease which could affect their sight, should not need sight tests more often than every 2 years".

The statement was issued as part of the process to protect public funds and to provide the "Health Authorities" in place at that time with guidance on when to look critically at the need for frequent sight tests. An increasing volume of sight test (GOS1) claims at short intervals between sight tests had been identified in some areas.

The effect of FPN713 was to increase the vigilance of Health Authority staff responsible for checking GOS1 claims in terms of frequency of sight testing and accuracy of submission. There was no attempt by the DoH to restrict early testing if it was considered clinically necessary by an optometrist. The main aim was to prevent early testing for non-clinical reasons such as when a patient had broken their spectacles or simply wanted a new "image".

As a result of increased vigilance and the new guidance the number of forms being returned to optical practices for clarification of reasons for early testing increased and this led to more work in the Health Authority, increased work in the practices, increased costs with postage and delays in payments to contractors. The increasing pressure created was identified by some Health Authorities and reviews were undertaken to see how the issue could be approached to reduce the problems. In Dorset for example in 1999 separate local guidance on what would be acceptable for early testing was agreed between the Health Authority and the Local Optical Committee (LOC) that reduced the workload for both Authority and practices (Dorset HA 1999). A review of how the newly introduced system affected practice activity was published subsequently by the Chair of the Dorset LOC (Bell 2000).

As local areas introduced guidance on claims it was decided by the DoH that to prevent a "postcode lottery" a national system was required and in January 2002 after discussion between representatives of the AOP, College of Optometrists, FODO and DoH a "Memorandum of Understanding" was introduced by the DoH. At the same time guidance on appropriate intervals between sight tests was included in the *Code of Ethics and Guidance for professional Conduct* produced by the College of Optometrists. The College guidance still contains information on frequency of eye examinations under sections A60 to A64 (College of Optometrists 2021).

Content of the Memorandum

The memorandum was essentially in 2 sections the first identifying intervals that were considered as clinical possibilities and the second a series of codes to identify reasons where a sight test was to be carried out at less than the identified options. To ensure compliance and prevent abuse the system was to be audited through a Post Payment Verification (PPV) process.

The scheme meant that Health Authority staff could accept GOS1 submitted claim forms that met the criteria and would only challenge forms that fell outside the recognised criteria reducing the checking workload significantly. Random audit checks via PPV would then be used to identify outliers in the system and would check patient records to ensure that clinical details included in the patient record supported the claim submissions. New GOS1 forms had been introduced that included a box requesting a code to be included where a sight test was at an interval of less than the options tabulated in the MoU document.

The document also re-inforced the use of clinical judgement by clinicians for selecting appropriate intervals between sight tests but expected an accompanying justification to be available on the patient record. It should be remembered that although 2 years has become an "accepted" interval by custom and practice this in terms of GOS is still a "minimum" and where there is no clinical need for a test the 2-year time scale may not be seen as appropriate. A 25-year-old patient with no prescription, no underlying health issues and no family history of eye problems could well be advised to have a longer interval between testing if this was considered appropriate.

The MoU was also clear in differentiating a GOS sight test from other services and where assessment or monitoring was being carried out as part of a co-management scheme and a diagnosis had been made in the secondary care sector GOS would not apply. In these cases, payment should be made from hospital or community health service funds. However, where refraction is required as part of an agreed protocol an NHS sight test may be appropriate for eligible patients.

Next appointment interval flexibility

The guidance also recognised that appointment making required some flexibility in practice — for example if the patient was going to be away for a holiday at the time their appointment would be due. It was therefore accepted that claims for a sight test carried out within one month of the expected retest date would not be challenged on receipt of the claim but again a justification for this early review should be noted on the patient record. Should it be found that this flexibility was being used more frequently than would be expected there was potential for an audit to be carried out.

Minimum intervals between sight tests

As mentioned above Section 2 of the MoU relates to *minimum intervals between sight tests* and the intervals were agreed as acceptable clinical possibilities. The document still however reiterates the requirement for practitioners to satisfy themselves that a sight test is necessary. It goes on to specify that the intervals included in the MoU should NOT be read as applying automatically to all patients in an identified category.

Table 1 shows the agreed minimum intervals included in the original MoU and the only subsequent interpretation amendment to these categories is for patients with Diabetes. Currently where a patient with diabetes is included as part of the National Diabetic Retinopathy Screening programme (introduced in 2003 and considered to have reached national coverage by 2008) a 1-year review on the basis of the diabetes is considered as unnecessary as the patient would be receiving a retinal assessment via imaging and therefore normal intervals apply.

This section provided information on the expected most frequent potential early sight test reasons. Any patients falling within one of these categories did not require a code and GOS claims for these patients would be approved automatically but would be audited during any PPV process to ensure the system was being used appropriately.

Table 1:   Minimum Intervals between sight tests from original MoU (2002)

Patient Age at Time of Sight Test or Clinical Condition	Minimum Interval Between Sight Tests
Under 16 years, in the absence of any binocular vision anomaly	1 year
Under 7 years with binocular vision anomaly or corrected refractive error	6 months
7 years and over and under 16 with binocular vision anomaly or rapidly progressing myopia	6 months
16 years and over and under 70 years	2 years
70 years and over	1 year
40 years and over with a family history of glaucoma or with ocular hypertension and not in a monitoring scheme	1 year
Diabetic patients	1 year

Patients outside specified categories

This provision of acceptable clinical reasons still left what was considered likely to be a small number of patients that did not fall within any of these categories or who required a sight test at an interval less than those provided in Table 1. To accommodate these patients section 3 of the MoU provided a selection of codes for *"Reasons for Earlier Sight Test"*.

The introduction to Section 3 confirms that a sight test may be carried out at a shorter interval than those listed in section 2 either:

- At the practitioner's initiative for a clinical reason or
- Because the patient presents him/herself to the practitioner with symptoms or concerns which might be related to an eye condition.

In these cases, the GOS1 form must be annotated with a specific code from the list for England in Table 2 and a record of the code used and the reasons should be included on the patient record for future PPV purposes. The coding is different in Scotland and Northern Ireland.

Table 2: Reasons for Earlier Sight Test according to the MoU

Code	Reason
1.	Patient is at risk of frequent changes of prescription for reasons not requiring medical referral or for reasons already known to a medical practitioner
2.	Patient has pathology likely to worsen, for example age-related macular degeneration, cataract, corneal dystrophy, or congenital anomalies.
3.	Patient has presented with symptoms or concerns requiring ophthalmic investigation
	3.1 resulting in referral to a medical practitioner; or
	3.2 resulting in issue of a changed prescription; or
	3.3 resulting in either no change or no referral (the patient's record should indicate any symptoms shown to support this category of claim, if necessary).
4.	Patient
	4.1 needing complex lenses; or
	4.2 with corrected vision of less than 6/60 in one eye.

(Continued)

Table 2:   (*Continued*)

Code	Reason
5.	Patient
	5.1 has presented for a sight test at the request of a medical practitioner; or
	5.2 is being managed by an optometrist under the GOC referral rules, for example suspect visual fields on one occasion which is not confirmed on repeat, or abnormal IOP with no other significant signs of glaucoma; or
	5.3 is identified in protocols as needing to be seen more frequently because of risk factors.
6.	Other unusual circumstances requiring clinical investigation.

Interpretation and Misunderstandings

The first major misunderstanding that arose, but which now seems mostly to have been resolved, was due to contractors failing to identify that the quoted intervals in Table 1 did not apply to **all** patients in a particular category. Despite the fact that it is very clearly set out in the document that each patient should be treated individually it was not followed. In some instances, reminder programmes were amended on computer systems to generate a letter for any patient in the recognised category at the minimum acceptable interval and not only those where the reduced interval between tests was clinically necessary. There are still occasions (after nearly 20 years of operating) where during Post Payment Verification checks of GOS sight testing this mistake is found on patient records.

The initial widespread use of reminders for all patients in a particular category led to some organisations caring for patients with visual problems promoting on their websites the need for regular testing at the reduced intervals. This in turn led patients to believe that there was an "entitlement" to have a sight test at the reduced interval or at most every 2 years. Even today there is some confusion over this with patients with no problems seeing recommendations advising a check every 2 years (or less in some instances) and believing they have an entitlement to at least a 2-year check. But this does not map on to the GOS contractor requirements where the clinician must satisfy themselves that a sight test is necessary.

The second area where misunderstanding and misinterpretation become apparent and remains today relates to sections 2 and 3 of the MoU. When it was written this part of the MoU was made less specific and designed to cover all eventualities. In achieving this however by specifying ophthalmic investigation the content blurs the lines between a sight test as defined by the Opticians Act (1989) and by the NHS GOS contract terms and wider examination of the patient. Section 36(2) of the Opticians Act defines sight testing as '*determining whether there is any and, if so, what defect of sight and of correcting, remedying or relieving any such defect of an anatomical or physiological nature by means of an optical appliance prescribed on the basis of the determination*'.

But further to this para 3(1) of The Sight Testing (Examination and Prescription) (No 2) Regulations SI 1989/1230 states that:

... when a doctor or optometrist tests the sight of another person, it shall be his duty —

(a) To perform, for the purpose of detecting signs of injury, disease or abnormality in the eye or elsewhere —

  (i) An examination of the external surface of the eye and its immediate vicinity,

  (ii) An intra-ocular examination, either by means of an ophthalmoscope or by such other means as the doctor or optometrist considers appropriate,

  (iii) Such additional examinations as appear to the doctor or optometrist to be clinically necessary.

One interpretation of the term "sight test" as defined in the Opticians Act has been taken as relating only to the assessment and correction of refractive error with the additional tests included once the need for a sight test has been determined seen as a form of eye health screening. The optical profession itself has sought to differentiate refraction from eye examination and the content of a sight test has been in discussion for a considerable time without agreement and this has again muddied the waters.

Pathologies

In the MoU the codes do not specify that the early sight test should only relate to a potential refractive change indeed if we look at Code 2 and take age related macular degeneration (AMD) as an example the clinical symptom most likely to be noted by a patient is reducing vision, but this is unlikely to be refractive. Does this therefore mean that such patients should not be seen within GOS, or could AMD be considered as an anatomical or physiological change? Does this fit with the GOS interpretation? The MoU in the introduction to this section introduces the phrase *"pathology likely to worsen"* but does not relate this to refractive change and there is an implication therefore that assessing vision change symptoms associated with pathology is part of GOS.

"Flashes and Floaters"

An example where interpretation has proved even more difficult is the case of flashes and floaters. Here there is a symptom or concern relating to an *"eye condition"* as noted in the MoU introduction that potentially is sight threatening but is most unlikely to be a refractive issue. Interpretation by NHS Areas has varied but in many cases Flashes and Floaters are excluded from GOS resulting in charges for private tests, the development of schemes or attendance at eye casualty when perhaps not necessary. Taking the MoU at face value the patient has presented with symptoms which might relate to an *"eye condition"* and under code 3 the concerns require an *"ophthalmic investigation"*, and one could by implication again expect this to be covered by GOS.

GP Referrals

A further example that may lead to misunderstanding is Code 5.1 *"the patient has presented for a sight test at the request of a medical practitioner"*. In some cases, GPs interpret this to mean that if they would like to rule out a visual/ocular issue then the patient can be sent to the optometrist in some instances solely for a check of Intra Ocular Pressures. This is a misunderstanding of the GOS system as applied by the NHS.

To oblige the GP and to be able to claim a GOS payment an Optometrist would have to complete a full sight test — however according to the NHS contract before carrying out a GOS examination the clinician must satisfy themselves that such a sight test is clinically necessary. Where no referral notes are available from the GP and in a patient that perhaps has been recently sight tested complaining of the same symptoms a GOS sight test would not be considered appropriate.

Catch-all

The final code in the table is Code 6 "*Other unusual circumstances requiring clinical investigation*". An interpretation of the term clinical investigation could lead one to believe that this was more than just a measurement of refractive error. According to the NHS Data Model and Dictionary: "*A Clinical Investigation is a clinical test or investigation offered to or carried out on a person it may include blood tests for specific antibodies, scans or physical examinations for specific diseases (NHS 2020).*"

It is clear how a misinterpretation could occur.

As a final contributing factor to misunderstanding the scope of practice of optometrists has expanded markedly since the MoU was first produced and there is much greater involvement in multidisciplinary care. Changes to the involvement by optometrists in ocular therapeutics has provided opportunities to become more involved in management of patients in different settings. A review undertaken by the AOP (Warburton 2013) indicated that the MoU was still considered reasonably effective concluding "*although practitioners propose sight test recall intervals to reflect the needs of each patient, the MoU nevertheless continues to reflect safe sight test intervals in the view of the majority of practising clinicians, just as it did when it was first introduced*" — however that review was published some years ago and the profession has developed rapidly in the intervening period.

In 2022 the MoU is being revisited and hopefully a new version will address the issues of interpretation and potential misunderstanding but with the continuing development of commissioned services and pressures on secondary eye care services clarification of the MOU is long overdue.

Chapter 4

Interpreting GOS Queries

In order to fulfil the GOS contract, providers and performers must comply with various guidelines and requirements that relate to the contract and have been established over time. Inevitably areas arise where clarity or interpretation is required and a guide to some of the most common issues that arise together with a reference to the source documents where the original guidance can be found is given below.

The advent of e-GOS creates additional issues and although most contractors are now linked to the system there are still some using paper hard copy processes and there are glitches within the electronic system that cause a contractor to revert to a hard copy. The regulation and guidance issued to cover hard copy processes is still in place but does not necessarily apply to the e-GOS situation and this will be an ongoing issue until all contractors are on the electronic system and guidance has been re-written accordingly.

Frequency of sight testing

Note FPN 713 issued in October 1997 states 'it is for optometrists and OMP's to decide how frequently a patient's sight needs testing'. It then goes on to state that in the view of the Department of Health adult patients with refractive errors, but no underlying disease or risk factors should not need a sight test more often than every two years. Although FPN 713 is still current a Memorandum of Understanding (MoU) was produced in 2002 after consultation between the DoH and professional bodies that expands on when testing at an interval of less than 2 years may be acceptable. Details of the MoU can be found in Chapter 3. From a GOS audit standpoint it is important that clinical records clearly identify reasons for early testing.

Previous sight test date

The date to be used on the GOS1 form indicating the date of the previous sight test must be the last sight test undertaken whether this was private, GOS or performed overseas. This means that the date of the last GOS test should only be used when no subsequent sight test has been performed.

Display of Notices

At each premises at which a contractor provides GOS services, the contract requires that a NHS England approved notice indicating the services available under the GOS and terms of eligibility for such services must be displayed prominently (SI1996/705).

Information must be available to patients about the complaint procedure operated within the practice and the details should include details of the person nominated within the practice to investigate and deal with complaints. This information should be displayed together with the alternative route available for complaints via NHS England. Where the complaint relates to GOS it should be indicated that should a patient be unhappy with the way their complaint has been handled there is an appeal route via the Health Service commissioner (Ombudsman). For complaints other than GOS i.e., relating to spectacles or contact lenses, if the practice is unable to deal satisfactorily with the issue details of the Optical Consumer Complaints Service should be available. (National Health Service Complaints [England] Regulations (2009) and the GOS Contracts Regulations (2008).

Small Frame Supplement

Introduced in 1997 this additional payment was intended to cover the situation in which a non-standard frame and lenses had to be produced at additional cost in which the datum centres were not more than 56 millimetres apart (or box centre distances of not more than 55 millimetres). The requirements were however changed in HSC 1999/051 when small frames became available as standards from stock. The new definition states 'small glasses means glasses for a child under 7 years who needs a custom made or a stock spectacle frame which requires extensive adaptation to ensure an accurate fit and has a boxed centre of no more than 55 mm. For this purpose, boxed centre is to be construed in accordance with Part 1 of BS 3521/91 (Terms relating to optics and spectacle frames) published by the BSI' as updated by British Standard BS EN ISO 8624:2011 (Ophthalmic Optics. Spectacle Frames. Measuring System and Terminology)

Examples of extensive adaptations are given as:

- Reductions or increases in the length of sides
- Manipulations to reduce or increase the bridge width which cannot be achieved solely by adjustment of the pads
- Lenses with a high, positive spherical power worked to minimum substance (either by the practice or a wholesale supplier).

Where exceptionally a patient of 7 or over requires small glasses, NHS England should be consulted. (NHS (Optical Charges and Payments) Regulations 1997, SI 1999/609 & HSC 1999/051)

In April 2016 the Optical Charges and Payments Regulations were amended (SI 2016 325) and accompanying guidance was introduced to allow a Special Facial Characteristics (SFC) supplement to be claimed by GOS contractors in Primary Care. The supplement is payable where a frame has to be custom made or specially adapted and it was agreed that frames designed with appropriate modifications should also attract the Special Facial Characteristics supplement.

Where the Special Facial Characteristics supplement is being applied, there must be a clinical need for the specialist frames and to ensure equity, these frames are available also via the Small Glasses Supplement (SGS). For this to happen the current requirement for SGS must also be met and the specialist frame must be provided for clinical need rather than style choice.

Prior to 1 April 2016, the Special Facial Characteristics supplement was restricted to Hospital Eye Service Departments and the advice change was introduced to make arrangements more convenient for patients and to reduce pressure on secondary care. There were initial problems however with the introduction of the supplement, and it did not fully become operational until 2019.

Tinted lenses

Under the GOS a tinted lens should only be prescribed if it is judged to be clinically necessary by the performer, tints for cosmetic purposes are not available under the GOS. It is acceptable to provide a photochromic tint where appropriate and clinically necessary as specified in HSC 1999/051. Anti-reflection coatings and ultra-violet blocking tints cannot normally be supplied under the terms of the GOS. For some patients undergoing dermatological treatment where there may be a risk to the eyes from UV light it may be possible to justify providing a UV filter under the HES regulations. Plano tinted spectacles for assistance in dealing with children with dyslexia are not covered within the GOS regulations. (FPN 713 and HSC 1999/051)

Non-Tolerance

If a second eye test is undertaken due to an intolerance of the prescription by the patient, then any new GOS form submitted should be annotated 're-test/non-tolerance' and coded appropriately. The same details should be entered onto the patient record. Having completed the test a new voucher cannot be issued without the prior approval of NHS England and a form is available normally to use when applying for a non-tolerance approval. If authority is given by telephone, then the Voucher should be annotated with the name of the person authorising and the date on which authority was given (FPN 713). Non-tolerance must relate to the prescription supplied to the patient and not to the lens form supplied and must not be as a result of an error in testing or recording.

Completing form GOS1

Once eligibility for a sight test has been demonstrated the details on the form should be duly completed. It is not necessary for the patient to complete the details, but it is necessary for the patient to sign the form to confirm the details are correct (SI1997/818). It is an offence to submit false or incorrect details and a patient may be liable to a penalty charge if found guilty of such an offence. When signing the GOS1 form the patient makes the following declaration: *I declare that the information I have given on this form is correct and complete. I understand if not, appropriate action may be taken against me including repayment of the NHS sight test fee and payment of a penalty charge.*

By 2021 most practices had moved where possible to the use of electronic GOS forms. The patient is still required to sign these to confirm details are correct and that requirements are understood.

Altering Prescriptions

Transposition

All prescriptions issued under the GOS should be written in the highest spherical power to provide for the optimum patient voucher value. If as a supplier a prescription is received that is not in this form, then it can be amended on the voucher and then the amendments initialled and annotated FPN:713 (FPN 713). The electronic system should automatically correct this error, but it is essential to ensure that is has been enacted.

In the case of a HES (P) form no changes can be made to the form in which the prescription is written even if transposition would prove an advantage to the patient by increasing the value of the voucher.

Back Vertex Distance (BVD) changes

Where it is found necessary to amend a voucher prescription to take account of BVD then the supplier should initial the changes and add 'BVD change'. If, however amending the prescription takes it to a higher Voucher band then the prescriber's authority to make the amendment is required. It would be necessary for the prescriber to amend and initial the voucher or to send a note or fax (email) authorising the change. (FPN 713) The removal of fax systems and the introduction of protected electronic systems for e-GOS should remove this as a potential problem.

Complex lenses

A complex lens is defined as a lens with a power in any one meridian of greater than plus or minus 10 dioptres or a prism controlled bifocal lens. Any patient requiring a complex lens is entitled to a NHS sight test and they may also be issued with a complex lens voucher unless they are entitled to a spectacle voucher on income grounds in which case, they cannot receive the additional amount for a complex lens. A patient entitled to a complex lens voucher would also be entitled to supplements for tints, prisms, or small frames where considered clinically necessary.

If a patient, previously requiring a complex lens is found during an NHS sight test to no longer require a complex lens they would still be eligible to receive an NHS sight test on this one occasion even though they do not meet the eligibility requirement. Also, anyone undergoing a private sight test who is found to require a complex lens during the test can be asked to complete a GOS1 switching the test to NHS. (FPN 713)

Small prescriptions and small prescription changes

Where a sight test results in a small prescription or small change that is considered clinically insignificant a voucher should not be issued other than when spectacles are to be replaced for fair wear and tear. (FPN 713) The College of Optometrists has issued general advice on what would constitute a clinically insignificant change of prescription, but a GOS PPV review would take each patient result on its own merits. If a small prescription is to be given a note indicating why the decision has been taken should be made on the patient record.

Lifetime of a prescription

The maximum lifetime of a prescription is 2 years and spectacles should not normally be made up to a prescription that is more than 2 years old (HSC 1999/051 and SI 1984/1778). Where a patient, for clinical reasons, at the end of their sight test is advised that an early retest is required then the life of the prescription issued is only until the advised retest date.

Issuing of a Voucher

An appropriate GOS 3 voucher should be issued at the time of the NHS sight test to all those eligible. In the case of a paper copy the patient should sign Part 1 of the GOS 3 form at the time of the test to confirm eligibility. The patient may take the voucher to any supplier legally able to provide them with an optical appliance. The patient should sign Part 2 of the form GOS 3 only upon receipt of spectacles (FPN 713). This situation is amended with the introduction of e-GOS as eligibility is checked electronically and access to a Voucher issued elsewhere can be via the electronic system. As the Voucher is stored on the system there is no need to provide a hard copy to the patient and therefore the signature process is amended.

Lifetime of a Voucher

Once issued unless an earlier sight test has been recommended a Voucher has a lifetime of two years to bring it in line with the maximum expected life of a prescription. In the case of an earlier test recommendation the Voucher has the lifetime of the earlier interval. Where there is a delay between issue of a Voucher and its use the patient must still be eligible for a voucher at the point at which they eventually use it for the Voucher to be valid to order spectacles.

Where a patient appeared to have lost a Voucher NHS BSA could authorise a practice to issue another if it was satisfied that the voucher had not already been used. This authorisation to issue a second voucher could be given to a practice that did not issue the original voucher. Any voucher issued in this way should have been annotated with the information and the name of the person giving authority and should carry the date on which the replacement was issued (SI 1999/609, HSC 1999/051, SI2013/461). However, the introduction of the e-GOS system means that this procedure is for the most part redundant as the required information as to whether a Voucher has been used or not will appear on the e-GOS system unless for whatever reason a paper version has been issued.

Submission of Vouchers

Vouchers for sight testing (GOS1 and 6) should be submitted to NHSBSA for payment within six months of the date on which the sight test took place. Vouchers for the supply of optical appliances or repair or replacement should be submitted within three months of the date on which the appliance was supplied, repaired, or replaced (SI1997/819). Although still in place the advent of electronic GOS systems should make these submission deadlines redundant as the submission process allows for direct electronic submission.

Change of Eligibility status

If a patient can show evidence of NHS eligibility following a private sight test and before ordering spectacles it is not necessary for them to undergo a second test. Instead, the supplier should complete a GOS 3 form and copy over the details of the private prescription (HSG (97) 48 & FPN 706) and submit with a covering note.

Where a patient has been issued with a GOS3 but becomes ineligible for a GOS3 before the Voucher is used then the Voucher becomes ineligible for payment.

Spare pairs of spectacles and repairs and replacements

No patient has been automatically entitled to a spare pair of glasses of the same prescription. Exceptionally — e.g., where a child with a disabling illness is breaking glasses with such frequency that education is being disrupted — permission may be sought from NHS England to allow supply of a second pair. In the case of permission for a second pair claims should be submitted on form GOS(V)/GOS(3) and the form annotated with the name of the person at NHS England who gave authority.

Where a second pair has been issued under the above arrangements the patient is automatically entitled to have either pair replaced or repaired provided that they are children using a GOS4 Voucher. Under GOS (General Ophthalmic Services) Regulations (Optical Payments and Charges Regulations 2013) SI 2013/461 adult patients who qualify for GOS can receive a repair or replacement voucher (GOS4) if they are eligible and NHS England has accepted the loss/breakage is due to illness. You should not repair or replace an adult's spectacles until confirmation has been received from NHS England indicating approval that the breakage or loss was due to illness and that the loss or damage would not have occurred but for that illness. In very exceptional circumstances of major hardship NHS England may consider replacement of stolen or broken spectacles without which the patient would have extreme difficulty in working (FPN 706 & FPN 713). Details of how to apply for an adult repair/replacement were provided at https://pcse.england.nhs.uk/media/2286/gos-4-pre-authorisation-briefing-v0-3-003.pdf.

In the case of supply of an appliance to a child by a hospital, repairs can be carried out as if the supply had been via GOS and claims made on a GOS 4 form. Where an adult is supplied with an appliance through the HES, they should be advised to consult the hospital in the case of loss or breakage. (FPN713)

If a patient has been tested and no change made to their spectacles, but spectacles are subsequently broken shortly after the test, where the optometrist judges that there was unlikely to have been any clinical change in prescription, a voucher could be issued on the grounds of fair wear and tear without a further examination. (SI 1999/609 & FPN 713). The interval between sight test and supply however should not be excessive.

High Reading Additions

To assist patients who may otherwise seek to apply for a low vision aid the voucher appropriate to bifocal spectacles is to be determined by the power of the reading add when it is greater than 4.00 dioptres more powerful than the distance prescription. For all other bifocal prescriptions, the voucher value is determined solely by the power of the distance correction. (HSC 1999/051)

Payments by instalment

If a patient opts to buy glasses by instalment but subsequently establishes eligibility for a refund of a voucher value no refund will be made until such time as the patient has paid instalments equivalent to the voucher value. (SI 1999/609 & HSC 1999/051)

Patient Refunds

A patient applying for a refund must establish their eligibility within three months of the date on which they paid for the glasses or, in the case of payment by instalment made the first payment. (SI 1999/609, FPN 706 & HSC 1999/051, SI2013/461)

Contact Lenses

A patient may use a GOS 3 voucher towards the purchase of prescription contact lenses, but the prescription written for spectacles should not be amended on the form to match the contact lens prescription. Where the contact lens prescription is in a higher or lower band than that for the spectacles the voucher value appropriate to the spectacles should be issued. A voucher for replacement of 'durable' contact lenses can be issued based on fair wear and tear if an optometrist judges them to be unserviceable. Within the terms of the GOS, contact lenses will be considered to be disposable if they require replacement at six monthly intervals or less. A voucher should not be issued for supply of further disposable contact lenses on the grounds of fair wear and tear and may only be issued based on a change of prescription at a valid re-examination. (FPN 713)

Where a patient loses or breaks a contact lens which is not defined as disposable within the GOS and is eligible for replacement (i.e., a child or an adult judged by NHS England to have lost or broken the lens through illness) a voucher for replacement spectacles should be issued. If the patient wishes this voucher can be put towards the cost of a replacement contact lens.

Varifocals

If a patient is supplied with varifocals as an alternative to bifocals, then a voucher may be issued, and the value claimed is as if bifocals had been supplied. (FPN 713)

Eligibility for a NHS Sight test relating to Glaucoma

Anyone undergoing treatment for glaucoma and anyone that has undergone surgery for glaucoma is entitled to a NHS sight test.

Any patient that has been referred to the ophthalmology department with raised IOP and suspect glaucoma and found clear but advised by the ophthalmologist to seek regular monitoring because they are at risk of glaucoma may be treated as eligible for NHS sight tests.

Parents, siblings, and children of patients in the above categories who are over 40 years of age are eligible for NHS sight tests. (FPN 713 & SI 1999/693)

However, where a patient is attending the HES for management of glaucoma the appropriate interval between GOS sight tests will be considered as not less than 2 years and the MoU to validate an earlier interval will not apply unless alternative clinical reasons for an earlier test are present.

Eligibility for a NHS sight test due to Diabetes

Once diagnosed patients suffering from diabetes are always likely to be at risk of diabetic eye changes and therefore should continue to be eligible for GOS. As with glaucoma patients however where a diabetic patient is being seen annually within the national Diabetic Eye Screening Programme the appropriate interval between tests would be considered as not less than 2 years unless alternative reasons for an earlier test are present.

Overseas visitors' eligibility to receive NHS GOS

The regulations relating to overseas visitor access to NHS services was amended by the National Health Service (Charges to Overseas Visitors) Regulations 2015 SI 2015/238. The result is that any organisation providing NHS funded services is required to make and recover charges to overseas visitors for services they have received unless they are primary care services (as set out in the NHS Act 2006) or an exemption applies. In 2018 NHS England issued updated guidance to NHS providers about how to implement these charges.

As far as GOS sight tests are concerned as these are primary care services, they are available to overseas visitors at no charge if they fall within the criteria for an eligible person as outlined in Chapter 2. This is consistent with the eligibility criteria established by the Primary Ophthalmic Services Regulations 2008 which include no nationality or residence requirements.

This eligibility does not extend to secondary commissioned services for which a charge would be made.

Student eligibility for GOS on age grounds

Students leaving school and continuing in education by starting at a university or college and who would be eligible for GOS on age grounds remain eligible between leaving school and starting university or college providing that they do not intend taking time out. Time out is considered as being when they do not intend to leave school and start further/higher education in the same calendar year. If they have left school and have a confirmed place for continuing education, they should enter in the appropriate section of the GOS forms the name of the university or the college they are due to attend. If the patient is awaiting confirmation of the place, then the school details should be used.

Reglazing spectacles

Where a patient whose prescription has changed opts to use an existing frame for reglazing Form GOS(V)/GOS3 should be completed and the appropriate voucher value or the cost of the reglaze, whichever is the lower, should be claimed. If only one lens is to be reglazed a claim for the voucher value or the private charge for one lens whichever is the lower can be submitted. There are no 'half' vouchers, and the full voucher value will be due if the normal private retail price for the supply and fitting of one lens exceeds the voucher value.

Where a prescription has changed in one eye only, but the patient requires a new frame the appropriate voucher value or the cost of supply of the new spectacles, whichever is the lower, should be claimed. (FPN713)

Point of Service Checks

Introduced in February 2001 a point of service check on eligibility must be carried out when a patient applies for a sight test on the NHS or a voucher for supply of an optical appliance is accepted. Where no evidence is available the GOS form should be marked accordingly. (GOS circular January 2001)

Domiciliary visits

When carrying out a domiciliary visit the patient must indicate the health problems that prevent them attending a practice. The patient or the carer will need to certify that they have requested a domiciliary visit, because of inability to leave home unaccompanied, by completing the appropriate box on the GOS form. Details of requirements are found in

The General Ophthalmic Services Contracts Regulations 2008 SI 2008/1185.

Mobile practices are required to register with NHS England where the business offices are situated and the host NHS England area where they intend to provide a domiciliary service.

Domiciliary Services to day centres are limited to those that provide for:

- Patients with disabilities who would otherwise require a sight test at home
- Children with special needs attending non-residential schools
- Members of ethnic communities unaccustomed to using mainstream health care facilities and who would be best served by receiving care in their community surroundings
- Genuinely homeless people of no fixed abode who are unlikely to be able to access services in a community practice.

Even when day centres fall within these categories patients to be eligible for GOS must be non-ambulant or incapable of accessing community optical practices without undue difficulty.

Chapter 5

The NHS and Complaints

Introduction

The National Health Service contract requirements for the provision of ophthalmic services were reviewed in Chapter 2. The aim of this chapter is to outline the NHS processes and most likely routes of action following receipt of a complaint against a contractor or performer. In practice there are two main processes that can be brought into play when a complaint is made the first process is patient driven and the second process is NHS driven.

It should be remembered that it is always better to deal with a complaint rapidly, before escalation and seek local resolution. When dealing with a patient complaint the suggested advice for a contractor would be:

- Keep as calm as possible
- Try to keep the patient as calm as possible
- If possible, move to a private area for discussion
- Listen carefully to the complaint and try to understand the patient's view
- Establish the facts and understand the complaint
- If unsure of your position do not make hasty decisions — offer to review the details of the complaint and get back to the patient
- Avoid admitting liability but remember the duty of candour
- Establish what action the patient is seeking

- In many cases it will be more cost effective, without admitting liability, to change a product or offer a goodwill refund than to have a protracted argument

NHS compliant process

The GOS contract requires a contractor to have in place a NHS regulation compliant procedure that acts as the first step in dealing with a patient complaint. This allows minor disagreements to be dealt with effectively within practice and avoids intervention by the NHS.

Contractors are required to meet specific standards and provide services as agreed (See Chapter 2) and in England it is the responsibility of NHS England to monitor the standards of service provision in their area. Should a contractor or practitioner not meet the required standard or breach the terms of the contract NHS England will take appropriate action. Similar processes apply in Northern Ireland, Scotland, and Wales.

The NHS complaints system in England

The NHS complaints system in England was revised by *The Local Authority Social Services and National Health Service Complaints (England) Regulations 2009 (Statutory Instrument 2009 No. 309)* that came into effect on 1 April 2009. The introduction of NHS England in April 2013 and a change to the OCCS complaints service in April 2014 led to minor modifications to the system.

Currently the system:

- Allows a patient to complain directly to the Director of Commissioning Operations (DCO) if they wish
- Requires contractors to record all the complaints received about GOS services, domiciliary sight-testing and locally commissioned community NHS services provided
- Requires the remedial actions taken and the lessons learned to be recorded

- Requires contractors to report annually to the NHS England DCO in their region the number and nature of all such complaints received and the important actions taken.

NHS guidance states that, for the purpose of operating the system, a complaint:

- must relate to GOS or a locally commissioned service only
- can include the process involved in the issuing of optical vouchers (but not the appliances supplied)
- is not a complaint, if it is made orally and is resolved by the practice within 24 hours
- is not a complaint, if it concerns dispensing services or spectacles or lenses which are entirely private arrangements.

As noted above all GOS contractors in England are obliged through the GOS contract to have in place arrangements to deal with complaints about services provided. This is a statutory and contractual requirement covering sight testing and the issue of prescriptions and optical vouchers but not dispensing of spectacles as this activity falls outside of the GOS. Where a contractor also provides commissioned NHS services normally these would fall within the same complaint requirements. The contractor is also required to display information about the complaints procedure and to have documentation available about the procedure to inform patients if requested (sample documents produced by the Optical Confederation are available).

Why have a consistent process established for complaints?

The arrangements for dealing with complaints are set up to ensure that:

- complaints are dealt with efficiently
- complaints are properly investigated

- complainants are treated with respect and courtesy
- complainants receive, so far as is reasonably practical —
  - o assistance to enable them to understand the procedure in relation to complaints; or
  - o advice on where they may obtain such assistance
- complainants receive a timely and appropriate response
- complainants are told the outcome of the investigation of their complaint
- action is taken, if necessary, in the light of the outcome of a complaint.

To achieve the above a contractor is expected to take responsibility for arrangements for dealing with complaints, designate an individual as the complaints manager, display information to inform the public of the arrangements in place and maintain a record of all complaints and submit these annually to NHS England. An electronic system is available for this process.

Normally a complaint should be received within twelve months of the incident giving rise to the complaint although in certain circumstances this period may be extended. A complainant may be a patient; or a person acting on behalf, and in the interests, of a patient; or a third party actually or potentially affected by the substance of the complaint.

A complaint about NHS services may be made directly to the practice involved or via the local DCO but a complainant cannot use both routes. If the complaint is made to NHS England, NHS England is obliged to consider it and can decide to handle the complaint itself. Alternatively, NHS England may, if it is considered appropriate and with the complainant's consent, refer the complaint to the practice for resolution. This latter course of action is recommended in most circumstances by Department of Health guidance.

What must a contractor do?

On receipt of a complaint a contractor must:

- acknowledge receipt of the complaint within three working days
- offer to discuss the complaint with the complainant. Whether or not the complainant meets the contractor or their representative the

contractor must inform the complainant about how the complaint is to be dealt with and how long it will take

- try to resolve the complaint within six months
- keep a record of all the complaints received and associated paperwork/ electronic documentation.

Records relating to complaints may be stored separately from patients' clinical records, although it would be a sensible procedure to cross reference in the clinical record that there has been a complaint.

Where investigation of the complaint takes a long time, efforts must be made to keep the complainant informed of the progress of the investigation. As soon as possible after an investigation is completed the complainant must be informed in writing of how the complaint has been considered and what is proposed to resolve the complaint and any consequent action. At this point the complainant should also be advised of their right to pursue the complaint with the Health Service Commissioner (the 'health service ombudsman') the final arbiter where resolution has not been possible.

Annual reporting of complaints

The annual report required of GOS contractors should be sent to the DCO and contain details of the number of GOS complaints received in the year in question, the number of complaints which were justified ('well founded') and the number referred to the ombudsman.

In the report the nature of the complaints received must be summarised providing information on any matters of general importance arising out of the complaints or the way in which they were handled, and any action taken to improve NHS services resulting from the complaints. An online system was established in 2019 to enable contractors to submit this annual data electronically. It should be remembered that the report is for public information and must be made available to anybody on request.

Where a complaint specifically states or implies negligence the advice is simply to acknowledge receipt of the complaint and to consult a representative body or insurance provider, before attempting to resolve the matter or admitting liability.

NHS investigation of a practitioner following a complaint

Whenever concerns are raised about the performance of a primary care performer or contractor (and this may be linked to a complaint for other reasons) there is the potential for the matter to have an impact upon patient safety or for it to impinge upon the wider public interest. In all cases where a concern is raised the NHS Commissioning Board (NHS CB) will evaluate the circumstances and associated risks to determine whether any immediate action is required in order to protect patients.

The duty to protect patients is of paramount importance and the priority in the NHS CB's performance procedure will be to assure and maintain patient safety and public protection. In these instances, care will be taken also to protect the performer or contractor, for example referral to occupational health services if appropriate.

Performance issues

In addition to contractors listing to provide GOS any optometrist who wishes to perform NHS sight tests in England must be included in NHS England's national ophthalmic performers list in accordance with the National Health Service (Performers Lists (PL)) (England) Regulations 2013. As most optometrists in England perform GOS sight tests they are bound by the performer list regulations that provide NHS England with powers over admission, suspension and removal from its lists and the responsibility for maintenance of the performers lists. The powers are there to enable NHS England to ensure that performers are suitable to undertake NHS primary care services and to protect patients.

A performance concern can relate to any aspect of a performer's conduct or performance and the concerns may arise from a variety of sources and may present themselves in various ways e.g., poor clinical performance, management or administration that may compromise patient care, a breach of professional boundaries with patients, colleagues or staff, non-compliance with professional guidelines or even criminal acts. There may be single or multiple underlying causes for under-performance, and it is the responsibility of the local Responsible Officer to ensure that any concern regardless of how minor is reviewed and, if required, acted upon promptly, fairly, and proportionately in accordance with the *The Medical Profession (Responsible Officer) Regulations SI 2010 No 2841* that came into effect on 1 Jan 2011.

Dealing with Performance issues

In fulfilment of its responsibilities NHS England in 2013 published a framework to deal with issues raised *The Framework for Managing Performance Concerns in Primary Care*. This was revised for implementation from 1st April 2015. The framework provides the overriding principles for how NHS England teams that support the Responsible Officer should discharge their statutory functions and ensures that concerns are handled in a way that protects patients and the public, maintains high standards and is consistent and fair to performers.

Performance Advisory Groups (PAGs) and Performers List Decision Panels (PLDPs) were set up within each Area Team and any complaint or concerns raised would in the first instance be dealt with by a PAG unless the issue was so serious that an immediate suspension from the performer list was considered necessary in which case a decision would be made by the medical director and one other director in the Area Team. However, this decision must be reviewed by two members of the PLDP who have not been previously involved in the decision to suspend, within two working days beginning on the day the decision was made. The case must then be considered by the PLDP to consider any representation received.

Performance Advisory Groups

A PAG was intended to offer expertise provided by individuals with in-depth knowledge of performance procedures and professional standards and able to provide advice on handling individual cases. Membership comprises of four voting individuals. These are:

- A senior NHS manager with a performance role who would chair the PAG

- A discipline-specific practitioner nominated by the medical director and in the case of an optometrist this would be either the Optometric Adviser or an appropriate individual nominated by the LOC
- A senior manager with experience in primary care contracting and/or patient safety and experience
- A lay member.

The first three members must be present for the PAG to be quorate. All members have a vote, and the chair has the casting vote, if necessary.

The PAG may request further fact-finding, e.g., a review of records before making decisions about any further action. Based on this and any other information available to the PAG it may decide:

- That there is no patient safety or public interest concerns and that no action is required.
- To manage the concern informally by agreeing a local action plan with the performer, and/or by a meeting with the performer and/or a recommendation for them to discuss the issues with their employer/mentor/appraiser.
- That there is need for a formal investigation before decisions about any further action may be taken.
- To refer/signpost the performer to their medical practitioner/occupational health if it involves a health issue before decisions about any further action may be taken.
- To arrange mentoring.
- To arrange a period of supervision.
- To refer the case to the Performers List Decision Panel (PLDP) to formally invoke the Performers List Regulations

Most concerns are resolved locally at PAG and closed without the requirement for any escalation. Research shows that the earlier a concern is identified and addressed, the more likely that a satisfactory and successful outcome will be achieved. It is important therefore to ensure that the process for identifying concerns is robust.

Performer List Decision Panels

The PLDP take overall responsibility for the management of performance, decide on actions required on individual performance cases in line with the Performers Lists Regulations and any other statutory regulations and make referrals to other bodies where appropriate. Cases are referred to the PLDP where:

- local resolution has failed to address the concerns, or
- it is deemed necessary to impose conditions, or
- there is a requirement to suspend the performer from the list, or
- there are significant patient safety/conduct issues, or
- there are serious performance/conduct concerns that have either
  i. resulted in serious patient harm or
  ii. may seriously undermine public confidence.

Membership of the PLDP comprises of the following individuals:

- A lay member who will chair the PLDP.
- A discipline-specific practitioner.
- A senior NHS England manager/director with responsibility for patient safety/experience.
- The Medical Director for an NHS England team or their nominated deputy.

All four members need to be present for the PLDP to be quorate. All members have a vote, and the chair has the casting vote, if necessary. Additional non-voting members and advisors may also be invited by the chair from time to time. In addition, the performer may be accompanied by a legal representative or an advocate or LOC member.

The PLDP will consider concerns referred to them by the PAG along with the supporting information provided and based on this may decide to:

- Take no further action.
- Refer back to PAG for further investigation or monitoring.

- Consider referral to the primary care contracts team for consideration under the relevant contract regulations.
- Agree an action plan for remediation of the performer when appropriate, including a reporting process for monitoring of the implementation of the action plan.
- Refer to the GOC.
- Refer to the police.
- Refer to NHS Protect.
- Take disciplinary action which results in conditional inclusion, contingent removal, suspension, exclusion, and removal.

The performer will have the opportunity for an oral hearing with representation and support, legal or otherwise, at the hearing. Having decided to invoke the Regulations and having given the performer notice of the proposed action, the PLDP, possibly in the form of an oral hearing panel, will then determine, dependent upon the grounds and evidence presented, what action, if any, should be taken.

Appeals to Tribunal

A performer has the right of appeal to the First-tier Tribunal Primary Health Lists if the NHS Commissioning Board (NHS):

- refuses to add them to a performers' list
- removes them from the list
- keeps, changes, or adds to the conditions of including them on the list

Appeals are considered by the First-tier Tribunal (Primary Health Lists) which is independent of the government and will listen to both parties. The tribunal will undertake a complete re-hearing of the case with evidence presented by the NHS and by the individual or their representative before reaching its decision. In the case of Optometry, the re-hearing panel will be made up of a judge, an optometrist, and a layperson with relevant health experience. The hearings are held in public and attended by a clerk or usher.

The Health Service Ombudsman

The Ombudsman service is a free service that will make final decisions on complaints that have not been resolved by the NHS in England and UK government departments and other public organisations. Any decision is taken fairly and without taking sides. As the ombudsman service is the final arbiter for unresolved complaints the expectation is that the complainant will have followed the normal complaints process of the organisation involved and that this has been exhausted without resolution of the complaint. This is to provide the organisation initially with the opportunity to examine the concerns raised and, where necessary, put things right.

The service has a three-step process for dealing with complaints. An investigation is the final step in the process and not all the complaints received reach this stage.

Once work on an investigation is completed and a decision made the decision is sent to the complainant, the organisation against whom the complaint has been made and any other person or organisation who was involved in the complaint. Occasionally reports are shared with other organisations, such as a regulator, where an organisation has been requested to make improvements to services which the regulator needs to keep a check on.

If recommendations are made for an organisation to implement, the Ombudsman's report will clearly explain what actions are expected and by when and this will be followed-up by the Ombudsman office.

Optical Consumer Complaints Service (OCCS)

Whilst not part of the NHS system the OCCS is a useful route for dealing with consumer issues in optics including those arising from the NHS. NHS England signpost patients to this service where complaints relate to spectacles provided or other consumer issues. Following the review of UK optical services by the Optical Services Audit Committee (OSAC) (see Chapter 8) one of the recommendations made was to establish an independent complaint service. This service was intended to cover all aspects of optical services and goods provided by registered optometrists and dispensing opticians. The result was the establishment of OCCS in

1992/3. Funding had been an issue since it was set up with initially ABDO, FODO and the Central LOC fund providing financial support, but the GOC took over the role of commissioning the service in 2005.

OCCS was not set up as a disciplinary body and should be viewed as an independent and free mediation service for consumers (patients) of optical care and the professionals providing that care. The service should not be seen as an alternative to a practice's internal complaints procedure where the majority of complaints are resolved. However, if a consumer and practitioner cannot resolve the complaint, either can refer the complaint to the Optical Consumer Complaints Service that will review the details and assist in finding a resolution. Where a practitioner fails to respond to a request from OCCS no further action can be taken other than to advise the patient on their rights and the processes remaining for them to pursue the complaint. It is advisable however for a practitioner to enter into dialogue if approached by OCCS.

If someone other than the patient makes a complaint on the patients' behalf written authority from the patient is required before the complaint can be registered. The OCCS although funded by the GOC from registration fees uses a firm of solicitors and is totally independent and impartial so that each complaint is considered fairly.

In the year to March 2019 OCCS received 1493 enquiries the majority of which (45%) related to goods and services with 35% relating to customer care. In the same period only 6% related to charges. Overall OCCS recorded an 87% success rate for completing enquiries through mediation.

Complaints to the GOC

NHS England may decide that a complaint contains information that requires involvement of the statutory body the GOC. In these circumstances the NHS can make a referral of the complaint. Sometimes referral will be following the outcome of a full NHS procedure but on other occasions it may be considered more appropriate for the GOC to deal with the complaint from the early stages and before the NHS investigation has begun.

The GOC has a process for reviewing all complaints received and dealing with them appropriately. The Fitness to Practice system of the GOC is discussed in detail in Chapter 13.

Non-NHS Complaints

As it is a contractual requirement to have in place a complaints process that is compliant with NHS requirements it is generally considered by most practitioners to be sensible to use the same format and timetable for any non-NHS complaints other than minor issues. Where a serious complaint is made about clinical or professional issues it is sensible to approach the appropriate professional organisation to seek advice. For example, both FODO and the AOP provide insurance services to cover such issues and will assist in dealing with complaints of a serious nature.

Complaints should not necessarily always be viewed in a negative light. By recording even minor complaints it can be seen if specific issues are being raised regularly and this can help to identify areas within the practice that may benefit from change or training.

Chapter 6

The Opticians Act

Introduction

The primary statute relating to optical professional practice in the UK currently is the Opticians Act 1989. This was a consolidated Act based on the original Opticians Act 1958 but incorporating the various amendments that had been introduced in the intervening 30 years. As a consolidating Act there was no intention to introduce any further changes to the legislation in place. There have been a significant number of amendments to the legislation since 1989 however and the most significant were via The Opticians Act 1989 (Amendment) Order 2005, made under Section 60 of the Health Act 1999, which came into effect with its supporting Rules on the 1 July 2005. This was one of a series of Orders that the Government made at the time to modernise the health care professions in the UK and significantly affected the provision of optometric and optical care and the framework within which the optical professions practise and optical businesses operate.

The amendments to the Opticians Act significantly improved the way in which the GOC could protect the public by bringing about changes that affected registration, recognition of specialties, professional indemnity insurance, continuing education and training, registrants' fitness to practise and contact lens supply.

How was the Opticians Act Developed?

In the introduction to this text the transition in optics in the UK from a company to professional bodies was outlined, the original body being the Worshipful Company of Spectacle Makers founded by Royal Charter in 1629 followed by the British Optical Association that was formed in 1895. The professional bodies continued to evolve, and the introduction of examinations ensured that by the early years of the twentieth century the profession was controlled, in terms of standards of training, by examination. Despite this progress, no legislation was available to endorse this activity. Members of the professional groups were very keen to see this situation changed and lobbied Parliament for the introduction of such legislation.

Hopes were raised of a successful outcome when the optical bodies gave evidence on the scheme for optical benefits to the Royal Commission which was established to consider the National Health Insurance Acts. Subsequently a Joint Council of Qualified Opticians drafted a non-prohibitive Bill for presentation to Parliament. The Bill was designed to provide recognition for opticians with an approved certificate or who had been in practice for at least 5 years before the introduction of this Optical Practitioners (Registration) Bill, and who had also passed a practical examination. The Bill was sponsored by Mr West Russell and received its first reading in February 1927 being passed for a second reading. Before the second reading could take place, the Ministry of Health instituted a departmental inquiry into the optical aspects of the Bill that effectively blocked any progress.

The Departmental Inquiry Committee consisted of three optometrists, three medical members, two members appointed by the Ministry and four lay members. The terms of reference for this committee were "to consider the optical practitioners (Registration) Bill and to make recommendations".

Towards the end of 1927 the committee published its report which proved a set-back for the aspirations of the optical profession. A majority report was signed by eight members, a first minority report by the three optometrists and a second minority report signed by an MP. The main stumbling block seemed to be the lack of consistency in training and standards set by the examining bodies with particular regard to the training and assessment in the recognition of ocular disease. The outcome of this was that the Bill was not resubmitted for consideration, and despite the majority report view that reconsideration would be possible, it was to wait until after the introduction of the National Health Service Act 1946, before this matter was again reviewed.

The Minister of Health in 1949 established an interdepartmental committee, under the chairmanship of Lord Crook, whose terms of reference were to advise on the assumption that it would be in the public interest that provision should be made by legislation for the registration of opticians, how registration could best be carried out, and what qualifications should be required as a condition of registration. The Committee itself consisted of 13 members, comprising optometrists, dispensing opticians, ophthalmologists, members of the medical profession, a physicist, a physiologist, a member of the teaching profession and a member of the general public.

Early in 1952, the Committee published a unanimous report in which they recommended that legislation should provide:

- For the establishment of a body to be known as the General Optical Council who would set up and maintain appropriate registers of optometrists and dispensing opticians.
- That all optometrists and dispensing opticians recognized by the National Health Service Act 1946 should be eligible for registration but that all future applicants would be required to possess a qualification from one of the recognized optical bodies.
- That the General Optical Council should exercise disciplinary powers over registered optometrists and dispensing opticians and have power to admit, remove and restore names to the registers and that they should maintain an appropriate ethical standard.
- That the General Optical Council should organize inspections of optical examining bodies and of the optical training institutions.
- That optometrists and optometry students should receive more training from medical men in certain subjects and be allowed to have further clinical training by medical men in appropriate hospital departments.

There were certain "special problems" the Committee considered during their deliberations which they felt were outside the basic terms of reference but were still worth noting. Within this category the following recommendations were made in the final report:

Corporate bodies.
Although there was no evidence to support the idea that corporate bodies were causing problems, the Committee felt that no new optometric bodies should be formed and that those already in existence should be allowed to continue at the discretion of the General Optical Council.

They also recommended that dispensing corporate bodies should be allowed to remain but that they should not involve themselves in any other activities and that a majority of their directors should be registered dispensing opticians.

Advertising.
This should be restricted and advertising relating to the refracting service should cease and that relating to dispensing services should be very limited. The recommendation was that the General Optical Council should review this area as a matter of urgency.

Co-operation between ophthalmologists and optometrists.
Hospital experience should be required of all those training as optometrists with the aim of providing links between practice and hospital to help foster a spirit of co-operation.

Recognition of ocular abnormality.
Registration of optometrists should not imply any ability to diagnose ocular or other diseases.

Orthoptics, contact lenses and use of drugs.
The General Optical Council should be given the task of reviewing each of these areas and be asked to make recommendations.

This set of recommendations was a marked step forward for the optical profession in public eye care, but despite pressure from many parties, the Ministers of Health failed, after repeated promises, to introduce legislation. It was not until 1957 that a bill presented as a Private Members Bill by the Member for Wembley South, a Mr Ronald Russell, was given its first reading. The Bill passed speedily through the Houses and received Royal Assent on 7 July 1958.

The Opticians Act 1958 (and subsequent developments)

According to the introduction to the Act the Opticians Act 1958 was:

"to provide for the registration of opticians and the enrolment of bodies corporate carrying on business as opticians; to regulate the practice of opticians and the conduct by such bodies corporate of their business as opticians; to impose restrictions on the testing of sight and the supply of optical appliances; and for the purposes connected therewith".

Within this framework a new body, the General Optical Council, was to be established to control registration and to make rules. The Act defined the testing of sight as:

"Testing sight with the object of determining whether there is any and if so, what defect of sight and of correcting, remedying or relieving any such defect of an anatomical or physiological nature by means of an optical appliance prescribed on the basis of the determination"

and went on to list those groups to which this function was restricted. The Act also:

- Restricted those able to be involved in the sale and supply of optical appliances.
- Prohibited the use of specified titles.
- Gave additional powers to the newly formed GOC to make rules prohibiting or regulating certain aspects of practice.
- Required the GOC to establish certain defined committees.

The Optician's Act Amendment Bill (1982)

Following the introduction of the Opticians Act 1958 there were pressures from commercial and political sources to alter some of the details of the Act. The restrictions of certain functions to be carried out only by qualified persons seemed to be against the general principles or interests of some groups, and this conflict let to two major developments. One of these was the Office of Fair Trading Report *Opticians and competition 1982*; the other, the attempted introduction of a bill, the Opticians Act (Amendment) Bill by Lord Rugby in 1982. It was Lord Rugby's contention that s.21 of the Opticians Act 1958 was too prohibitive. It states that:

> *"Subject to the following provisions of this section, a person shall not sell any optical appliances unless the sale is effected by or under the supervision of a registered medical practitioner or registered optician."*

Taking up the case put forward by an American company that wished to sell spectacles "over the counter" and without the need for eye examination or qualified fitting, Lord Rugby suggested that it was in the public interest to have this open market approach. The major public advantage seems to have been seen as the cost of such spectacles. The proposal received support from some quarters, and it is strange how the issues which had so rapidly carried through the original 1958 legislation (i.e., the advantages of screening and adequate qualified eye care) were now seen by some as totally unnecessary when, in terms of volume of patients and pressure on hospital services, the ophthalmic profession was probably even more in demand. The legislation passed its first reading and was given a second airing in the House of Lords on 18 February 1982. At this stage, when it was likely that the bill would have been defeated if it had gone to vote, Lord Rugby withdrew the paper because of the Government inquiry being undertaken by the Director General of the Office of Fair Trading.

Health and Social Security Act 1984

The Office of Fair Trading published its report, *"Opticians and Competition"* in December 1982. The report concluded that although opticians did not make undue profits there were certain measures that would, in the opinion of those producing the report, improve the service to the public. The main improvement would be by the introduction of competition into the supply of spectacles through removal of the professional "monopoly" on spectacle supply. Coupled with this, greater freedom to advertise would offer a wider choice and greater information to the public considering spectacles.

The Government took the Office of Fair Trading report as the basis for drawing up a bill with far greater scope than had been anticipated. In fact, the Health and Social Security Act 1984 had such far-reaching consequences that many of the organizations that had campaigned so vigorously for change now campaigned against the proposed legislation. The Act as a whole, was designed to amend or supplement existing legislation regarding optical services and the optical profession but also included changes to:

- The status and constitution of Family Practitioner Committees.
- Finance within the Health Service.
- Disablement allowances.
- Social Security benefits.
- Occupational pension schemes.
- Membership of Social Security appeal panels.

The eye examination service was left untouched by this legislation on the grounds that a necessary service of screening was met by optometrists. On the other hand, the legislation covering the supply of spectacles and the regulations governing the practice of optometry and the provisions of the Health Service were radically altered.

Health and Medicines Act 1988

Despite the radical changes introduced by the Health and Social Security Act 1984, there were still groups dissatisfied with the progress made and the extent to which the Opticians Act 1958 had been amended. Notable again among those calling for further change was Lord Rugby. The government was again under pressure to review financing within the National Health Service, and in line with its stated philosophy of freedom of the marketplace and removal of professional self-regulation, the time was ripe for a further change.

The government in 1986 produced a "blue-paper" entitled *"Primary Health Care: An Agenda for Discussion"*. The general ophthalmic services took only two pages of the report and discussed the success of the removal of the opticians' "monopoly" and reinforced the importance of the free NHS sight-test stating, *"The sight-test can identify health problems as well as a need for spectacles, so it is important that skilled sight-testing should remain readily available"*. The document also laid the foundation for the introduction of a voucher system to replace the NHS range of frames and lenses.

When the Health and Medicines Act appeared in 1988, in addition to removing the previous right of any individual to apply for an NHS examination contrary to the text of the 1986 "blue-paper", it amended certain sections of the Opticians Act 1958. The amendments related to s.20 dealing with restrictions on the testing of sight, supply of optical appliances and the use of titles and descriptions and tackled s.21 again which dealt with restriction on sale and supply of optical appliances.

The Opticians Act 1989

It became apparent that the many changes in Health Service legislation subsequent to the Opticians Act 1958 had made that Act very difficult to use and therefore, changes relating to optometrists and dispensing opticians were consolidated into a single Act, The Opticians Act 1989. The new consolidated Act replaced the 1958 Opticians Act as the principal statute relating to optometry in the UK and took account of amendments introduced through:

- The Criminal Procedure (Scotland) Act 1975
- The National Health Service Act 1977
- The Criminal Law Act 1977
- The National Health Service (Scotland) Act 1978
- The Supreme Court Act 1981

- The Health and Social Security Act 1984
- The Companies Consolidation (Consequential Provisions) Act 1985
- The Health and Medicines Act 1988

The Opticians Act 1989 was not, therefore, intended to introduce any new legislation, but simply pulled into a single statute all relevant Acts and orders relating to the provision of optometry services in the UK since the original Act of 1958.

The parts of the revised Act covered:

- The General Optical Council
- Registration and Training of Opticians
- Disciplinary Procedures
- Restrictions on Testing of Sight, Fitting of Contact Lenses, Sale and Supply of Optical Appliances and Use of Titles and Descriptions
- A general section Miscellaneous and Supplementary

General Optical Council (For a detailed review see Chapter 7)

The Act outlined the revised membership and constitution of the GOC that had developed over time and in addition to a Registrar, the Council by January 2002 was constituted as laid down in SI1998/3117 as follows:

- Nine persons nominated by the Privy Council, one of whom will be Chairman.
- Six persons chosen to represent registered optometrists.
- Five persons chosen to represent registered dispensing opticians.
- Four persons nominated by the examining bodies as follows:
  o Two nominated by the British College of Optometrists;
  o One nominated by the Association of British Dispensing Opticians, after consultation with the training institutions, who shall be a person engaged in the education and examination of persons training as dispensing opticians;

o   One who is a person engaged in the education or examination of persons training as optometrists and nominated jointly by the optometric training institutions.

• Four registered medical practitioners.

Members of the Council were to be appointed for a period of 5 years.

Registration and training of opticians

The primary task of the General Optical Council under the 1958 Act was the establishment of registers of qualified opticians. These registers were to be maintained by the GOC whose role was to:

• Control applications for registration.
• Require notification of changes in the particulars shown in the lists.
• Prescribe an annual fee for registration.
• Register additional qualifications.
• Refuse to enter or maintain a name if a registration fee was not forthcoming.
• Record the death of registered opticians.
• Publish annually either registers and lists, or amendments to the existing register.

Initially five registers/lists were published, and they related to:

• Optometrists who both test sight and fit and supply optical appliances.
• Optometrists who only test sight.
• Dispensing Opticians.
• Bodies Corporate carrying on business as optometrists.
• Bodies Corporate carrying on business as dispensing opticians.

The registers/lists were to contain name, address, approved qualifications, and any other details that may be prescribed.

Registration remains a requirement although there are now only 3 main lists:

- Optometrists
- Dispensing Opticians
- Bodies Corporate.

To be entered on to one of the registers, a person is required to satisfy the General Optical Council that they meet the requirements as given in s.8 of the Opticians Act 1989. A person may not, however, be entered in more than one register even if they possess the qualifications that would entitle them to be included in more than one. In addition to the original registers, student optometrists and student dispensing opticians are now required to register with the GOC (although this is under review) and lists of registrants with additional specialist qualifications are also available.

The approval of training institutions and qualifications and the supervision of training institutions and qualifying exams were also within the remit of the General Optical Council.

Disciplinary proceedings

Part 3 Sections 14 to 23 of the 1989 Act dealt with disciplinary procedures and sections 14 to 16 of the Act outlined the disciplinary proceedings and penalties for failing to meet the professional standards expected of a practitioner or Body Corporate and defined the various disciplinary orders available at the time as either:

- An erasure order under which the name of a registered optician or an enrolled body corporate can be removed from the relevant register.
- A suspension order under which registration of a registered optician or enrolment of an enrolled body corporate may be suspended for a period not exceeding 12 months. During such suspension the optician or enrolled body corporate will be treated as unregistered even though their name may still appear in the register and the registrar of the General Optical Council will monitor such suspension.

- A penalty order which would require the registered optician or the enrolled body corporate against whom the order had been made to pay a specified sum to the General Optical Council up to a maximum set in regulation.

The disciplinary process was completely revised by the 2005 amendment and introduction of a new system of Fitness to Practise. The GOC in support of these changes was given the role of establishing, maintaining, and providing guidance on standards of conduct and performance for registrants, whether individual, student or business.

In addition, the GOC were required to develop and keep under review effective arrangements to protect members of the public from registered optometrists, registered dispensing opticians and student registrants whose fitness to practise or, in the case of a student registrant, fitness to undertake training, is impaired. The process will be looked at in more detail in Chapter 13.

Restrictions on Testing of Sight, Fitting of Contact Lenses, Sale and Supply of Optical Appliances and Use of Titles and Descriptions

Testing of sight

Part 4 of the Opticians Act has had the greatest impact on the optical professions — this Part relates to "Restrictions on testing of sight, fitting of contact lenses, sale and supply of optical appliances and the use of titles and descriptions". Offences within this section are considered criminal in nature and although action may be taken by trading standards officers or the police it is normally the GOC who would seek to enforce the law.

The first section (s24) states "... a person who is not a registered medical practitioner or registered ophthalmic optician shall not test the sight of another person". The definition of testing of sight has formed the basis of many discussions but in section 36 subsection (2) of the Act it is defined as *"testing sight with the object of determining whether there is any and, if so, what defect of sight and of correcting, remedying or relieving any such defect of an anatomical or physiological nature by means of an optical appliance prescribed on the basis of the determination"*.

The development of new equipment and skills for the optometry profession has led to much debate over the differences between an eye examination, an eye test, and a sight test. In law however the only defined process is as shown above for a sight test and the other terms, although much used, have no legal basis.

The Act confirmed the testing of sight definition given in the Opticians Act 1958 and specified that the function was restricted to:

- Registered medical practitioners
- Registered optometrists
- Medical students
- Persons training as optometrists exempted under GOC rules

It is a criminal offence for an individual who is not registered in the optometrist register or registered as an ophthalmic medical practitioner to pretend they have registration. If found guilty of this offence a person could be given a fine not exceeding level 5 on the standard scale (in 2020 this was £5000).

Following the Health and Medicines Act 1988, and subsequent statutory instruments including SI1989/1230 an additional section was incorporated into the Opticians Act 1989 which detailed the duties to be performed on sight testing and certain provisions for action following the testing of sight. Section 26, therefore, of the new 1989 Act specified the requirements. It is a legal requirement for the examination to be performed adequately including such examinations of the eye for the purpose of detecting injury, disease, or abnormality in the eye or elsewhere as the regulations may require. Immediately following the sight test a written statement should be issued containing the particulars specified by the Secretary of State and indicating that an adequate examination was carried out and that referral is or is not required. In addition, a signed written prescription or if no prescription is needed a note to that effect must also be issued.

It is an offence to require a patient, as a condition of undertaking the sight test, to purchase any optical appliance that may be necessary from a specified person. It is also an offence to require payment of a fee prior to the testing of sight of any individual and the fee is only payable where the required duties have been met.

Failure to comply with these requirements has been considered as serious professional misconduct.

Contact lenses

Section 25 of the Act identifies those who are legally entitled to fit contact lenses. Once again it is a criminal offence for an individual to fit contact lenses when they do not appear within the specified lists of those legally qualified to undertake fitting. Any case for contravention of this would be taken to court and if proven the individual would be liable to a fine up to the specified maximum level 5 as quoted above. Regulation relating to contact lenses is covered by Chapter 11.

Sale and Supply of Optical Appliances

The Health and Social Security Act 1984, and the Health and Medicines Act 1988, both made amendments to the regulations regarding the sale and supply of optical appliances. These were incorporated into s. 27 of the Opticians Act 1989, which states that except for "excluded sales":

> *"a person shall not sell any optical appliance unless the sale is effected by, or under the supervision of a registered medical practitioner or registered optician."*

An "excluded sale" was subsequently defined as:

> *"a sale for a person not under the age of 16 of spectacles which have two single vision lenses of the same positive spherical power not exceeding 4 dioptres where the sale is wholly for the purpose of correcting, remedying or relieving the condition known as presbyopia."*

Any person contravening these requirements was liable to conviction and a fine.

A further sections (s27) within part 4 of the Act deals with the sale and supply of optical appliances. This was restricted to registered practitioners until the 1984 Health and Social Security Act opened up the situation to allow for supply of spectacles under specific conditions by a much wider grouping. This was followed by the legalisation of the sale of "ready readers" providing they were to specific parameters.

The Opticians Act specifies that any sale or supply (other than for "ready readers") must be effected against a written prescription issued by a registered medical practitioner or ophthalmic optician (optometrist) following a testing of sight by that individual. The supply against a written prescription must be within the time specified on the prescription with a maximum of two years as defined by SI 1984/1778. Any appliance supplied must conform to the relevant British Standard. In relation to "ready readers" the sale must be for a person who has attained the age of sixteen and the appliance must have two single vision lenses of the same positive spherical power not exceeding 4 dioptres. The sale of the appliance must be wholly for the purpose of correcting, remedying, or relieving presbyopia.

It is a criminal offence to supply an optical appliance in contravention of the current legislation and if found guilty of the offence a fine up to a maximum level 4 can be applied (in 2020 this was £2500).

Use of Titles

The use of recognized titles that were restricted was dealt with under s. 28 of the 1989 Act, and this stated that:

> *"any individual or, where appropriate, body corporate, shall be liable on conviction to a fine if he:*
> - *Takes or uses the title of ophthalmic optician or optometrist when not registered in either of the registers of ophthalmic opticians.*
> - *Takes or uses the title of dispensing optician when not registered in the register of dispensing opticians.*
> - *Takes or uses the title of registered optician or enrolled body corporate when not registered in any register.*
> - *Takes or uses any name, title, addition or description falsely implying registration in any of the registers.*
> - *Otherwise pretends to be registered in any of the registers."*

Miscellaneous and Supplementary

Section 31 of the 1989 Act outlined additional powers for the General Optical Council enabling the Council to make rules prohibiting or regulating the following:

- The use of publicity by registered opticians and enrolled bodies corporate in respect of the practice or business of optometry or dispensing optics but not restricting the display of optical appliances.
- The use of business names other than those under which individuals are registered or corporate bodies enrolled.
- The use of drugs by registered opticians, enrolled bodies corporate and their employees in the course of practice or business.
- The practice of orthoptics.
- The prescription, supply and fitting of contact lenses and the requirements to be allowed to prescribe, fit, or supply contact lenses.
- The referral of patients found to be suffering from an injury or disease of the eye.

Overseeing aspects of the GOC, Section 33 provided the Privy Council with the power to direct the GOC to carry out functions in a particular way and with a particular timescale if it appeared to it that the GOC had failed to carry out a function that was necessary. If the Council failed to comply, then the Privy Council was able to carry out the specific function. This default power did not apply to:

- The Constitution and functions of the Council.
- Qualifications for registration.
- The approval of training institutions and qualifications.
- The supervision of training institutions and qualifying examinations.
- Certain aspects of the disciplinary procedures.
- The allocation of monies that the Council may have available.

The Opticians Act 1989 (Amendment) Order 2005

Where the 1989 Act had been a consolidation of existing regulation, fundamental changes to the aspects of optometry listed below were introduced to the 1989 Act by The Opticians Act 1989 (Amendment) Order 2005. This became the definitive version of the Opticians Act and continues to provide the basis for the current position. This Order was introduced under section 60 powers included in the Health Act 1999 and was part of the government drive at the time to modernise health care professions in the UK. Although there have been several subsequent changes this was the last major change to the Opticians Act to date. The amendments made by the 2005 order covered

- the GOC (see chapter 7)
- registration including the registration of students
- recognition of specialities
- professional indemnity insurance requirements (see Chapter 17)
- continuing education and Training (see Chapter 9)
- fitness to practice processes (see chapter 13)
- contact lens supply (see Chapter 11)

The Opticians Act 1989 (Amendment) Order 2005 came into effect with its supporting Rules on the 30 June/1 July 2005. This was one of the series of Orders that the Government made to modernise the health care professions in the UK and as mentioned above significantly affected the provision of optometric and optical care and the framework within which the optical professions practise and optical businesses operate.

The amended Opticians Act was intended to improve the way in which the GOC can protect the public by bringing about changes that affect registration, recognition of specialties, professional indemnity insurance, continuing education and training, registrants fitness to practise and contact lens supply. It redefined the role of the GOC as the overseer of "*professional education, conduct and performance among registrants*".

The corner stone of the Opticians Act 1989 remained the General Optical Council established by the original 1958 Opticians Act. It is one of 13 organisations in the UK known as health and social care regulators. These organisations oversee the health and social care professions by regulating individual professionals and registered businesses. The GOC has responsibility for regulating the optical professions in the UK and currently deals with the registration of around 30,000 optometrists, dispensing opticians, student opticians and optical businesses.

The amendments introduced by SI 2005/848 were to be overseen by the GOC and the Statutory Instrument included powers for the GOC to review its structure.

The GOC retained four core functions:

- Setting standards for optical education and training, performance, and conduct.
- Approving qualifications leading to registration.
- Maintaining a register of individuals who are qualified and fit to practise, train or carry-on business as optometrists and dispensing opticians.
- Investigating and acting where registrants' fitness to practise, train or carry-on business is impaired.

Registration including the registration of students

As noted above Part 2 of the 1989 Opticians Act relating to Registration and Training of Opticians required the GOC to maintain registers of suitably qualified individuals or corporate bodies carrying on business as either dispensing opticians or ophthalmic opticians. Three registers and two lists were established by the 1958 Act and maintained in 1989, This position changed to the current position below with SI2005/848. In addition to replacing the term ophthalmic optician with optometrist the following registers were established:

- A single register for optometrists (combining the previous 2 registers into a single register)
- The register for dispensing opticians was retained
- For the first time two student registers were established one for students undertaking a qualification in optometry and one for students undertaking a qualification in dispensing optics.

To be included on any of these registers individual applicants need to satisfy the GOC that they meet the requirements laid down in sections 8 or

8A of the Opticians Act. An additional clause was incorporated via SI 2005/848 to cover potential overseas registrants particularly from the European Economic Area and European Union. Providing the GOC is satisfied that an individual has a right to practise in the United Kingdom as an optometrist by virtue of the European Communities (Recognition of Professional Qualifications) (First General System) Regulations 2005 or as a dispensing optician by virtue of the European Communities (Recognition of Professional Qualifications) (Second General System) Regulations 2002, and is a fit person to practise as an optometrist or a dispensing optician then they should be included in the appropriate register.

In addition to the changes to the registers described above the listing of corporate bodies under section 9 of the Opticians Act also changed. The two lists representing ophthalmic businesses and dispensing businesses became a single register of bodies corporate carrying on business as an optometrist or a dispensing optician or both. Also, the terminology was adjusted, and the term "registered optician" was replaced with the term "registered optometrist or registered dispensing optician".

As part of the registration changes it became a criminal offence to gain registration by pretending to hold a qualification that would enable registration.

Training

Part 2 of the 1989 Act laid down procedures for establishing and monitoring standards for initial training and qualification for all registered optometrists and dispensing opticians in practice in the UK. The 1989 Act enabled the GOC to approve training institutions offering instruction in optometry and in dispensing optics. Following on from this the final award from the institution had to be approved and recognised by the GOC in order for an individual to join the relevant register. As part of their role in maintaining standards of training the GOC were also required to publish lists of approved institutions and qualifications. The area of training was developed by the 2005 amendment order (see Chapter 7) to include areas of specialisation and how such qualifications should be recognised.

Recognition of Specialties

As the profession developed offering additional clinical services and specialist qualifications became available changes were incorporated through the 2005 Amendment to enable the GOC to determine which if any specialist qualifications should be permitted for inclusion in the register. See Chapter 7 for more detail.

Professional Indemnity Insurance

Although it had always been advised as good practice to have adequate professional indemnity insurance the 2005 Amendment introduced this as a requirement for continued registration. Registrants are required to confirm to the GOC at renewal that adequate insurance is in place. This measure was introduced to protect patients and ensure that should there ever be a problem with care adequate funding would be available to meet a patient's needs.

Continuing Education and Training

Once qualified prior to 1995 there was no drive for the optical profession to undertake continuing training to develop or simply maintain a level of knowledge and skill. A voluntary CET scheme was piloted and developed by the College of Optometrists initially in 1995 and by 2000 much of the profession were participating. This was not acknowledged by the Opticians Act 1989, and it was the Amendment to the Opticians Act in 2005 that introduced compulsory CET for optometrists and dispensing Opticians. The GOC had decided that this was essential to maintain the up-to-date skills and knowledge needed to practise safely and effectively.

More recently the need for CET/CPD has been extended to cover specialties and has provided a form of revalidation to meet wider changes in clinical regulation. More details can be found in Chapter 9.

Fitness to Practice

The disciplinary procedure was overhauled as mentioned above and a new Fitness to Practice procedure put in place providing additional powers and greater accountability. Establishing and operating these new processes was the remit of the GOC and details can be found in Chapter 13.

Also, in keeping with developments elsewhere a clause was incorporated into the 1989 Act by the 2005 Amendment enabling the GOC to take advantage of technology and increase its use of electronic documentation and electronic storage of information.

Contact lens supply

The 1958 Act did not contain any specific provisions regulating the sale or fitting of contact lenses. The 1989 Act inserted amending legislation and Section 25 of the 1989 Act provided that only registered medical practitioners and registered opticians may fit contact lenses, with specific exceptions for medical students and persons training as opticians. The Act did not however go beyond this, and it was the 2005 Amending order that developed contact lens regulation.

The amending regulations (2005) changed the term "registered optician" in the 1989 Act to registered optometrists and registered dispensing opticians. In addition, they introduced a definition of "fit" that requires anyone fitting a contact lens to provide the patient on completion of the fit with a signed written specification for each lens that would enable the lens to be replicated. The specification provided must have an expiry date and the fitter also must provide instructions and information on the care, wearing, treatment, cleaning, and maintenance of the lens.

The sale and supply of contact lenses was affected significantly by the regulatory amendments in 2005.

Non-registered suppliers were able to sell a contact lens to a person over the age of 16 years where the seller had:

- the original specification;
- a copy of the original specification verified with the person who provided it; or
- an order from the purchaser, submitted either in writing or electronically, which contains the particulars of the specification of the person who intends to wear the contact lens ("the wearer"), and the seller verifies those particulars with the person who provided the specification;

- the seller is reasonably satisfied that the goods ordered are for use by the person named in the specification;
- the sale is made before the expiry date mentioned in the specification;
- the seller is, or is under the general direction of, a registered medical practitioner, a registered optometrist, or a registered dispensing optician; and
- the wearer is not, so far as the seller knows, registered as sight-impaired or severely sight-impaired

The GOC made rules under Section 31 of the Opticians Act 1989 regulating the qualifications required by registered opticians before they may fit contact lenses. The regulation of the fitting of contact lenses appeared adequately provided for but for a variety of reasons the regulation of the sale of contact lenses still lacked real teeth. There was no specific regulatory reference in the 1989 Act to the sale of contact lenses and the Act does not include a definition of a contact lens. Contact lens regulation is dealt with in greater detail in Chapter 11.

Sale and supply of optical appliances

The 2005 Amendment provided an extension of the exemptions to sales of an optical appliance by including the sale of an optical appliance intended for use as protection or cover for the eyes in sports if:

- neither lens fitted to the appliance has a positive or negative spherical power exceeding 8 Dioptres;
- the appliance is an appliance with a single vision lens or single vision lenses;
- the appliance falls within any category of appliance specified in an order made by the Privy Council for the purposes of this section.

Protection of titles

Subsequent to the Opticians Act 1989 as amended by SI 2005/848 and The European Qualifications (Health and Social Care Professions) Regulations 2007 (S.I. 2007/3101) the titles optometrist, registered optometrist, dispensing optician and registered dispensing optician are protected. It is an offence to pretend to have a specialty or proficiency that qualifies for entry in the appropriate specialty register or to take or use any name, title, addition, or description falsely implying registration in any of the registers or pretend to be registered in any of the registers.

In addition, it is an offence for any student to pretend to be registered as a trainee optometrist or dispensing optician when they do not appear in the student register.

There is protection for optical business and any body corporate which:

- takes or uses the title of ophthalmic optician, the title of optometrist, the title of dispensing optician or the title of registered optician when it is not registered or
- takes or uses any name, title, addition, or description falsely implying that it is registered or
- otherwise pretends that it is registered

is liable on summary conviction to a fine of an amount not exceeding level 5 on the standard scale (in 2020 up to a maximum of £5000).

There is a special exemption from the above in cases where a registered optometrist or a registered dispensing optician dies or becomes bankrupt at a time when they are carrying on business or are in practice. For three years after death or bankruptcy (or longer if allowed by the GOC) in certain cases where the business is to continue under the same name the title may still be used. In the case of death this would be use of the name and title by:

- the individual's executors or administrators;
- the individual's surviving spouse or surviving civil partner;
- any of the individual's children; or
- trustees on behalf of
  o a surviving spouse or surviving civil partner or
  o any of the individual's children.

In the case of bankruptcy where a registered optometrist or registered dispensing optician becomes bankrupt at a time when he is carrying on business or is in practice as an optometrist or dispensing optician, an appointed trustee in bankruptcy may take or use in relation to that business or practice the name and any titles that could be used immediately before the bankruptcy.

However, where this process is followed and an offence is committed by the business relating to the testing of sight, fitting of contact lenses or the sale and supply of optical appliances the Fitness to Practice committee may, if they think fit, direct that the exemption should cease to apply in relation to that business or practice.

Offences by Bodies Corporate

In the case of bodies corporate the 2005 amendment specified that where a body corporate is found guilty of an offence under the Opticians Act any "responsible officer" of the body found to have connived or through neglect caused the offence will also be considered guilty. "Responsible officer" means any director, manager, secretary, or other similar officer of the body corporate, or of a branch or department of the body corporate, or any person purporting to act in any such capacity.

Action under the terms of the Opticians Act

As stated at the outset the Opticians Act forms the basis for the statutory regulation of the professions of optometry and dispensing optics in the UK. It is a mixture of criminal and professional statutes that apply to anyone involving themselves in the testing of sight and the supply of optical appliances. The GOC acts as the controller of standards and would be the body that would take action as necessary should failure to comply with the Act be identified.

Previous actions have been taken against individuals or businesses that have:

- carried out eye examinations when they do not appear in the relevant register
- supplied spectacles to a minor when not appearing in any of the relevant registers.

- supplied contact lenses direct to the public in breach of the requirements.
- failed to comply with the Act by not providing a copy of the patient's prescription at the end of the examination.
- asked the patient to pay a fee prior to an examination being carried out.

Conviction for a criminal offence

Many of the cases considered by the GOC relate to individuals who have been found guilty of criminal offences. The spread of these cases is wide ranging from sexual offences to causing death by dangerous driving and from fraud to misleading advertising. The route is there for the GOC to follow up on <u>any</u> conviction in a court for a criminal offence.

Criminal offences prosecuted by the GOC against non-registrants

The GOC has a role in maintaining regulation not only amongst registrants but also in ensuring that non-registrants do not commit offences in breach of regulations. Such breaches are considered criminal offences and examples of the type of breach are shown in Table 1

The GOC recently published the document Illegal Practice Protocol (2022) outlining the offences and processes that would be used to determine if a criminal offence had been committed and whether a private prosecution would be appropriate and how this would be prosecuted. The intention is that the guide ensures the GOC is proportionate, targeted and consistent in its approach to illegal practice.

Table 1: Criminal offences affecting non-registered persons

1. Pretending to have the required qualifications to enable registration with the GOC
2. Pretending to appear in any of the registers maintained by the GOC when not qualified to so appear
2. Use of any of the titles protected under the Act
3. Supply of spectacles or contact lenses (other than "ready readers") without a valid written prescription
4. Fitting of contact lenses when not having the appropriate qualification
5. Testing eyes when not appearing in the relevant register

Chapter 7

The General Optical Council

As described in Chapter 6, the fundamental outcome of the Opticians Act 1958 was the establishment of the General Optical Council (GOC) the statutory regulatory body for the optical professions that is responsible for the registration of optometrists and dispensing opticians. It is one of 13 organisations in the UK known as Health and Social Care regulators, these organisations oversee the health and social care professions by regulating individual professionals. The GOC regulates the optical professions in the UK and currently registers around 30,000 optometrists, dispensing opticians, student opticians and optical businesses. In line with the Opticians Act the GOC has four core functions:

- Setting standards for optical education and training, performance, and conduct.
- Approval of qualifications leading to registration.
- Maintaining a register of individuals who are qualified and fit to practise, train or carry-on business as optometrists or dispensing opticians.
- Investigating and acting where registrants' fitness to practise, train or carry-on business is impaired.

Background and Composition of the GOC

The 1989 Act provided the following revised membership of the GOC:

(a) six persons nominated by the Privy Council;
(b) six persons chosen to represent registered ophthalmic opticians;
(c) three persons chosen to represent registered dispensing opticians;
(d) six persons nominated by the examining bodies mentioned in this Schedule; and
(e) six registered medical practitioners.

This was amended in 1999 and again in 2002 following The General Optical Council (Membership) Order of Council 1998 (SI1998/3117) resulting in the following membership

(a) nine persons nominated by the Privy Council;
(b) six persons chosen to represent registered ophthalmic opticians;
(c) five persons chosen to represent registered dispensing opticians;
(d) four persons nominated by the examining bodies mentioned in this Schedule; and
(e) four registered medical practitioners. The four registered medical practitioners on the Council were ophthalmologists nominated by the Royal College of Ophthalmologists and one of the four a person appearing to the College to be a suitable person to represent ophthalmologists practising in Scotland.

This membership however was further amended following the introduction of The Health Care and Associated Professions (Miscellaneous Amendments) Order 2008 and membership became much more fluid. The amendment reads:

"The Council shall consist of—
(a) registrant members, that is members who are registered optometrists or registered dispensing opticians; and
(b) lay members, that is members who—
    (i) are not and never have been registered in a register, or a director of a body corporate registered in a register, maintained by the Council, and
    (ii) do not hold qualifications which would entitle them to apply for registration in one of the registers maintained under section 7 or 8B.

(2) *The members of the Council shall be appointed by the Privy Council.*

(3) *The Privy Council shall ensure that, at any time, at least one member of the Council lives or works wholly or mainly in each of England, Scotland, Wales and Northern Ireland.*

(4) *Before the Privy Council gives a direction to the Appointments Commission under section 60(1) of the Health Act 2006 to exercise any function of the Privy Council relating to the appointment of members of the Council, the Privy Council shall consult the Council."*

This paved the way for a dramatic simplification of membership that was determined finally by the Health Care and Associated Professions (Opticians) The General Optical Council (Constitution) Order 2009 SI2009/442 and this simply states: *"The Council shall consist of 6 registrant members and 6 lay members"*. The membership of council in 2022 is in line with this format.

Committees of the GOC

The Opticians Act 1958 and the Opticians Act 1989 both required the General Optical Council to establish specific committees. Currently there are five statutory committees of the GOC as defined under the Opticians Act and related Rules:

- Education Committee
- Companies Committee
- Standards Committee
- Investigation Committee
- Registration Committee

In addition, there are 3 non-statutory committees constituted in line with good governance practice:

- Audit and Risk Committee
- Remuneration Committee
- Nominations Committee

There is one further committee the Fitness to Practise and Registration Appeals Committee populated by independent hearings panel members. Although appointments are made through a process established by the GOC this committee has to function independently of the GOC. For further information see Chapter 13 on Fitness to Practise.

Structure of Committees

Following the original 1958 Act there were significant regulatory changes to the GOC committee structures and to the membership of GOC committees e.g., The General Optical Council (Committee Constitution Rules) Order of Council 2005 SI2005/1474. However, the changes to the GOC constitution that came into effect in 2009 following new legislation (The General Optical Council (Committee Constitution) (Amendment) Rules Order of Council 2008 SI2008/3113) required a complete revision of all the committee structures. At its meetings of 19th May 2008 and 3rd July 2008, the Council agreed the constitution of its statutory committees under the revised constitutional arrangements, and this resulted in the Membership as shown in Table 1.

Briefly the statutory committees are reviewed below:

Education Committee

The Education Committee was established under the terms of the Opticians Act 1958 as an advisory committee to the General Optical Council on all matters relating to optical training and examinations. The main functions were seen as advising the Council on the promotion of high standards of professional education of optometrists and dispensing opticians and on the supervision of training institutions and the qualifying examinations. Currently membership consists of a minimum of nine and a maximum of 18 individuals and of this number at least 3 are optometrists, 2 dispensing opticians, 3 lay persons and 1 registered medical practitioner.

The function of this committee has changed little since 1958 and its current role is to advise the Council and other committees on optical

Table 1. GOC statutory committee membership

	Education Committee	Standards Committee	Investigation Committee	Registration Committee	Companies Committee
Size	Minimum 9 Maximum 18	Minimum 9 Maximum 18	9 Members	Minimum 7 Maximum 14	11 members
Membership	At least: 3 optometrists 2 dispensing opticians 3 lay persons 1 registered medical practitioner	At least: 3 optometrists 3 dispensing opticians 2 lay persons 1 registered medical practitioner	3 optometrists 2 dispensing opticians 3 lay persons 1 registered medical practitioner	At least: 2 optometrists 2 dispensing opticians 2 lay persons 1 responsible officer from a business registrant	(Rule 6) 1 optometrist 1 dispensing optician 1 lay person 1 registered medical practitioner (Rule 7) 7 members who are not members of the Council and who represent the interests of business registrants
Quorum	5 including: 1 optometrist, 1 dispensing optician 1 lay person	5 including: 1 optometrist, 1 dispensing optician 1 lay person	5 including: 1 optometrist, 1 dispensing optician 1 lay person	3 including: 1 optometrist, 1 dispensing optician 1 lay person	A total of 4 2 under Rule 6 2 under Rule 7

training, education and assessment including the approval of training establishments and qualifications. It reviews the content and standard of education including the CET/CPD scheme recommending changes as considered necessary. It has been instrumental in developing and implementing the details of the Education Strategic Review that started in 2015 and was implemented in 2022.

According to the GOC the review was aimed at:

- *Recognising that the optical professionals of the future will need to have sufficient agility to navigate and thrive in a technologically dynamic environment and potentially changeable business models in a way that is safe, competent and meets patient needs and expectations.*
- *Balancing educational innovation and flexibility with the ability to achieve a consistent level of educational attainment, based on adequate assessment and supervision, that provides public assurance in the practice of the 'safe beginner/ starter', and segueing coherently into specialised postgraduate education and continuing training.*
- *Attaining and maintaining consistency of mechanisms to demonstrate readiness to join the register, by implementing educational quality assurance mechanisms that are cost-effective, proportionate and command public and professional confidence.*

The Companies Committee

The role of this committee (established by the 1958 Opticians Act) is again advisory and is to offer advice and assistance to the Council on all matters (other than investigation/fitness to Practise) relating to bodies corporate carrying on business as ophthalmic or dispensing opticians.

The Committee currently consists of eleven members appointed via different routes. The appointments include (in line with Rule 6) one registered optometrist, one registered dispensing optician, one lay person, one registered medical practitioner and (appointed under Rule 7) seven members selected from persons who are not members of the Council and who represent the interests of business registrants. The quorum of the

Companies Committee is four and must include at least two members of the Committee appointed under rule 6 and two members of the Committee appointed under rule 7.

Standards committee

The Standards Committee advises and gives assistance to the Council on the standards of conduct and performance expected of current and potential registrants. The committee consists of a minimum of nine and a maximum of eighteen members of which at least three are registered optometrists, three are registered dispensing opticians, two are lay persons and one is a registered medical practitioner.

Investigation committee

This committee has the function of investigating allegations relating to impairment of fitness to practise or in the case of a student impairment of fitness to undertake relevant training. The committee decide whether an allegation should be referred to the Fitness to Practise Committee, and if not, what the next course of action should be. The committee is made up of three registered optometrists, two registered dispensing opticians, three lay persons and one registered medical practitioner."

Registration committee

The Registration Committee advises the Council on registration issues, including the rules governing registration and publication of the registers. Currently it consists of a minimum of seven and a maximum of fourteen members and at least two are registered optometrists, two are registered dispensing opticians, two are lay persons and one is a responsible officer.

Registration

Currently the GOC is required to maintain a series of registers relating to registered optometrists, registered dispensing opticians, registered students and to keep a list of corporate bodies involved in the provision of optometry services, dispensing optical services or both. To be included on any of these registers individual applicants need to satisfy the GOC that they meet the requirements laid down in sections 8 or 8A of the Opticians Act.

In relation to students in training it is important that the patients that they examine should receive the same protection as they would have if they were seeing a registered qualified practitioner. The 2005 amendment to the Opticians Act 1989 obliged the GOC to create and maintain an entirely new register of students undergoing training in Optometry or Ophthalmic Dispensing, whether full-time, part-time, or by distance learning and whether in college, university or as pre- registration gradu-ates. Under the requirements of the amendment and subsequent regulation (The General Optical Council (Registration Rules) Order of Council 2005 SI 2005 No. 1478) students must register with the GOC before commenc-ing their training. This ensures that the training they receive and their patient contact during the training period falls directly under the control of the GOC. They will in addition be subject to the same requirements (except for the requirement of professional indemnity cover) as all other registrants and will face the same sanctions should their conduct fall below that expected by the GOC of a registrant.

For registered optometry students the term "training" covers the period of study at an "approved training institution" and the pre-registra-tion period up to successful completion of the PQE's (the pre-registration training may be within the training Institution and the process is currently under review).

An additional clause was incorporated to the Act via SI 2005/848 to cover potential overseas registrants particularly at that time from the European Economic Area and European Union. Providing the GOC is satisfied that an individual has a right to practise in the United Kingdom as an optometrist and is a fit person to practise as an optometrist (or a dispensing optician) then they should be included in the register. To sat-isfy itself of suitability the GOC would need to ensure that a person apply-ing holds a qualification as an optometrist or as a dispensing optician granted outside the United Kingdom, has had adequate practical experi-ence in the work of an optometrist or a dispensing optician; and is a fit person to practise as an optometrist or a dispensing optician. The Council may also consider if appropriate that to satisfy the conditions the person be required to pass additional qualifications/tests.

A single listing of business registrants superseded the separate registers of corporate optometrists' and of corporate dispensing opticians. It now includes all corporate bodies which operate in the UK using the titles or descriptions listed in Section 28 of the Opticians Act 1989 ("optometrist", "dispensing optician", "optician", etc.).

Retention of registration is annual and to meet the requirements for retention registrants must show evidence of having completed the required CPD, have adequate insurance cover in place, make declarations about their health and any criminal or disciplinary proceedings and pay the appropriate fee.

Overseas qualifications

The General Optical Council reviews all overseas qualifications to determine whether they are similar in subject matter and standard to the UK qualifications and whether holders of an overseas qualification should be allowed on to the GOC register. Only the qualification in Eire currently is accepted as equivalent automatically although this may change following recent changes to reciprocity and the UK leaving the European Union.

Many overseas qualifications do offer a standard and content adequate to be considered for partial recognition but do not necessarily provide the scope of experience expected of registrants. If, therefore, a person comes to the UK as the holder of a qualification given partial recognition, they will be expected to comply with imposed GOC requirements and succeed at examinations as prescribed by the General Optical Council and provide evidence of achieving an adequate standard at English before being granted permission to register to practise in the UK.

The GOC recognised the European Diploma in Optometry and Optics (accredited by European Council of Optometry and Optics (ECOO) and introduced in 2000) as a route to registration for non-UK applicants, however this qualification does not grant direct entry to the register. It is not an Approved Qualification under the Optician's Act and therefore Candidates who have passed the European Diploma will only be eligible for registration with the GOC, provided that the Council is satisfied they have demonstrated a satisfactory scope of clinical practice, and they are proficient in the English language.

The supplementary examinations are carried out currently by the College of Optometrists and normally include a general oral including legal aspects of practice and a practical examination covering a routine eye examination together with such additional papers as deemed necessary.

Changes to the status of overseas professionals since the UK withdrawal from the EU is likely to have some impact on this aspect over time.

The GOC's role in training

The Opticians Act originally provided the Council with the tasks of granting, where appropriate, the status of "approved training institution" for new training providers and regularly reviewing the status of existing already approved institutions. It also provided for a qualification to become an "approved qualification" if it appeared appropriate. Since 2005 in addition the role has been extended to include Continuing Education and Training (CET — rebranded as Continuing Professional Development or CPD from 2022) for registrants (The Opticians Act 1989 (amendment) Order 2005 SI2005/848 and The GOC (CET Rules) 2005 SI2005/1473).

For registered optometry students in 2021 the following were approved as training institutions by the GOC:

Anglia Ruskin University
Aston University
University of Bradford
Cardiff University
City University of London
Glasgow Caledonian University
University of Huddersfield
Plymouth University
University of Central Lancashire
University of Manchester

Teesside University
University of Hertfordshire
University of Highlands and Islands
University of the West of England
Ulster University

Portsmouth University had originally received provisional approval, but the course was suspended in 2019.

The GOC is required to appoint visitors whose role is to attend approved institutions and qualifying examinations and report findings back to the GOC as a way of maintaining standards. Where the GOC decides that an institution is no longer providing adequate training it can demand remedial action and can even remove recognition of the qualification from the institution as happened in the case of the Portsmouth university course. There is a right of appeal process to the Privy Council who, if after consultation, think fit may reverse the decision.

In addition to its undergraduate responsibilities the GOC has responsibility for ensuring that pre-registration supervision is adequate and that pre-registration examinations carried out on its behalf are to the required standard.

To support the training and to comply with the terms of the Opticians Act defining those entitled to test sight, the Council has made regulations for exemption to accommodate those training to become optometrists and other relevant groups. These can be found in SI 1994/70 and subsequent amendment SI 1999/2897.

Following the Education Strategic Review completed in 2021 the GOC introduced a new framework for providers of undergraduate training. This moved the emphasis towards outcomes and matching to the Standards of Practice rather than prescriptive numbers of events. It is recognised that the adaptation and development will not be immediate particularly for those well-established providers of undergraduate training and this is seen as a 5-year development to be completed by 2025. The changes also bring the pre-registration training year under the auspices of the University sector that will be required to ensure adequate and appropriate training in preparation for the pre-qualifying examinations.

Continuing professional development — CET/CPD

Although voluntary CET had been encouraged for some time it was following amendment to the 1989 Opticians Act that in 2005 the GOC introduced compulsory CET requirements via The General Optical Council Continuing Education and Training Rules 2005 (SI 2005/1473). These were rapidly amended (after one attempted submission was not approved by the Privy Council) by The General Optical Council (Continuing Education and Training) (Amendment No2) Rules Order of Council 2006 (SI2006/2901). The result was that approved CET was to be undertaken by registrants in 3-year cycles with a minimum of 12 CET "points" achieved for each year of the cycle giving a total of 36 points for each cycle. Registrants who had an entry in the register relating to a specialty were required to obtain 18 additional specialty points in the 3-year cycle giving a total requirement of 52 points per cycle.

The rules also contained details of action should a registrant fail to attain the required level of points in a cycle. By the 21st of January in the year following the end of the cycle in which the shortfall occurred the GOC registrar would serve notice on the registrant informing them of the shortfall and warning that failure to make up the shortfall by the 15th of March in that year would mean their name may be removed from the register on the 1st of April. Removal of a name from the register meant that a practitioner could no longer be entitled to work as an optometrist and test patients. In the case of a specialty registration failure to achieve the required points would mean that the specialty details may be removed from the register and the registrant would no longer be able to claim the specialty.

The requirements for CET providers and how the system was to be administered was also established at this time.

The Rules were reviewed in 2012 and as a result amended again through The General Optical Council (Continuing Education and Training Rules) (Amendment) Order of Council 2012 (SI2012/2882). These new rules specify several competencies (as determined by the GOC) that are required to be achieved during the 3-year cycle and introduce a requirement that half of the required points should be interactive points and half general points. For this purpose, interactive is where an event:

(a) requires physical attendance;

(b) is part of a supervised course of education and training; or

(c) is to be conducted by way of instantaneous electronic communication with one or more persons qualified as an optometrist or dispensing optician.

One further change brought in by this amendment is to require attendance at least once during a 3-year cycle at a peer review/discussion event. This would be an approved event which is conducted by way of discussion between the person undertaking the event and one or more persons qualified as an optometrist or dispensing optician.

The rules relating to shortfall were also amended by this order and the registrar was to notify the registrant 2 months before the end of the 3-year cycle that if no further events were undertaken by the end of the relevant period, the registrant would have a shortfall in CET requirements and may be removed from the register at the end of that period. This removed the previous 3 month "grace" period between January and April when additional points could be achieved and affirmed a 3-year cycle timescale.

Further amendments to the rules relating to CET became effective for the 3-year cycle commencing January 2022. The Rules change the description Continuing Education and Training (CET) to Continuing Professional Development (CPD) in line with other professions and amend the competencies from clinic specific areas to broader "domains". In addition, following the development of Zoom based sessions during the 2020 pandemic these are set to continue alongside the traditional formats for education provision. There is no change proposed to the "points" or the interactive requirements. CET/CPD is discussed further in Chapter 9.

GOC Rules on referral

Special reference was made in the Opticians Act 1958 to the need for rules to be formulated relating to disease or injury to the eye. This duty has been carried forward into s. 31 (5) of the Opticians Act 1989, which states:

> *'The Council shall make and submit to the Privy Council rules providing that where it appears to a registered optician that a person consulting*

him is suffering from an injury or disease of the eye, the optician shall,
except in an emergency or where that person is consulting him for the
purpose of being given treatment under rules 'relating to orthoptics' or
in such other cases as may be prescribed, being cases in which it is,
owing to special circumstances, impracticable or inexpedient to do so,
take the prescribed steps to refer that person to a registered medical
practitioner for advice and treatment.'

The original General Optical Council Rules were embodied in SI1960/1936 and remained unchanged until the latest 1999 revision (SI 1999/3267 The General Optical Council (Rules relating to Injury or Disease of the Eye) Order of Council 1999). These rules incorporated several minor amendments that had a significant effect on Optometry. The main disadvantage of the original rules was that as practice and clinical skills developed and optometrists were better able to identify abnormalities and monitor/manage minor conditions the rules prevented them from using the skills. As optometrists were not allowed to manage patients their only course of action in law was to refer — failure to do so meant they were effectively breaking the rules. If, however, they had referred every patient that was seen who presented with an abnormality the Hospital Eye Service would have been unable to cope. The result was that most practitioners with the tacit approval of other eye care specialists took a pragmatic approach to the rules. The 1999 modifications took account of the situation and legitimised the custom and practice status that had developed. In the longer term this has led to the development of co-management schemes in many areas of England and more extensive care systems established by the devolved administrations of the UK. In addition, the advent of supplementary and independent prescribing has led to greater optometry involvement in eye care and improved patient management services across the UK.

The current GOC Rules on referral as amended by The General Optical Council (Injury or Disease of the Eye and Contact Lens (Qualifications)) (Amendment) Rules Order of Council 2005 SI 2005 No. 1476 cover the following:

If a patient attending a registered optician appears to be suffering from an injury or disease of the eye, of which the patient's general medical practitioner may be unaware, then a report of any findings should be sent to the GP.

When referring, the following procedure should be followed:

(a) Advise the patient to consult their medical practitioner.
(b) Wherever possible, send to the registered medical practitioner named by the patient a written report of findings indicating the grounds for thinking that injury or disease of the eye is present.
(c) If action appears urgent, then such measures as are available to inform the general medical practitioner immediately, e.g., telephone, shall be taken.

A patient cannot be forced to accept a referral and if a patient who appears to be suffering from injury or disease of the eye is unwilling, on conscientious or other grounds, to consult a registered medical practitioner, the optometrist should record that fact and the grounds which the patient gives for unwillingness to consult a registered medical practitioner.

If in the professional judgement of an optometrist or dispensing optician there is no justification to refer or referral would be impracticable or inexpedient then the clinician may decide not to refer but, in this case, should:

- record a full description of the injury or disease noted
- give the reasons for deciding not to refer
- record details of any advice or treatment given to patient
- if appropriate and with the consent of the patient notify the GP of the action and reasons.

Exception to duty to refer to medical practitioner

As an exception to the duty to refer to a registered medical practitioner, a registered optometrist may refer a patient who appears to be suffering from injury or disease of the eye to —

(i) a person other than a registered medical practitioner who provides and who has the appropriate qualifications or expertise to provide medical or clinical treatment for the injury or disease of the eye from which the person appears to be suffering, or

(ii) a person or body one of whose functions is to refer or to organise the referral of persons who appear to be suffering from an injury or disease of the eye to a registered medical practitioner or a person falling within sub-paragraph (i) if satisfied that the referral to that person or body is appropriate in the circumstances of the case.

However, where a registered optometrist makes a referral under part (i) of this exception the following details should be recorded on the patient record:

- details of the person consulting
- that the referral has been made and the date of the referral,
- a sufficient description of the injury or disease from which that person appears to be suffering, and
- details of any advice or medical or clinical treatment tendered to the patient.

In addition, the person to whom the referral is made should be provided with a written report of findings indicating

- the grounds for thinking that the person may be suffering from injury or disease of the eye;
- the urgency of the case

If the referral is made using part (ii) above it should include instructions as to whether the patient should be referred to a registered medical practitioner or a person who is not a registered medical practitioner, in which case the instructions should include the qualifications or expertise that person must have.

A further exception to the duty to refer applies to a registered optometrist who has the supplementary prescriber specialty and is acting under and in accordance with article 3B of the Prescription Only Medicines (Human Use) Order 1997 SI 1997/1830 or an optometrist who has the independent prescriber qualification.

None of the regulations regarding referral prevent an optician from rendering in an emergency whatever services are in the best interests of the person consulting.

These rules by the General Optical Council place a greater duty on the registered optician to refer a patient than do the NHS contract requirements. Under the NHS contract where an optometrist feels that further investigation is required then the patient's GP should be notified, and the patient referred. Where the clinician feels it more appropriate for them to monitor the situation then the patient's GP should be informed of this.

What is included in an assessment at a sight test?

The rules laid down in SI 1989/1176 (The Sight Testing (Examination and Prescription) Regulations 1989) also affect investigation for disease and injury and complement the General Optical Council Rules. They are made under the Terms of s. 26 (1) of the Opticians Act 1989 and are incorporated as an amendment to the Opticians Act 1958 imposed by the Health and Medicines Act 1988. The requirement in s. 3 (1)(a) of SI 1989/1176 is that it shall be the duty of a doctor or optometrist testing the sight of another person to perform for the purpose of detecting signs of injury, disease, or abnormality in the eye or elsewhere:

- An examination of the external surface of the eye and its immediate vicinity.
- An intra-ocular examination, either by means of an ophthalmoscope or by such other means as the doctor or optometrist considers appropriate.
- Such additional examinations as appear clinically necessary.

Rules on publicity

The General Optical Council made its first rules on publicity in 1964 and these were the source of much debate in subsequent years, particularly following the Office of Fair Trading Report (1982) and the efforts of Lord Rugby to introduce "ready readers" into the optical market. It was suggested that there should be relaxation of the publicity rules to allow wider freedom to advertise and thereby, in theory, increase competition. Further pressure was placed on the General Optical Council with the introduction of the Health and Social Security Act 1984, which allowed a wider marketing of spectacles and opened-up competition to both registered and unqualified suppliers.

At this time the General Optical Council submitted amended Rules to the Privy Council, but these were not found acceptable to the Privy Council on the grounds that the proposed Rules were still too restrictive. Previously the Rules would have been returned to the General Optical Council for further modification but using the powers granted under the Health and Social Security Act 1984 the Privy Council drew up and imposed their own set of regulations that were, after formal agreement by the General Optical Council, issued as SI 1985/203.

Under the terms of these amended rules a registered optician or an enrolled body corporate could use publicity in relation to practice or business providing that:

- It was legal, decent, honest, and truthful.
- It did not bring the profession into disrepute.
- It did not contain any reference to the efficiency of facilities provided by other registered opticians or bodies corporate.
- Any claims made were capable of substantiation.
- No claims were made suggesting superiority over any other practice or business.

The changes in regulations prompted a dramatic increase in the number of registered practitioners prepared to advertise. The type, style and quality of advertisements were inevitably variable, and it must be said that many advertisements came extremely close to breaking the regulations. The wider use of advertising agencies with an open brief led to some registered opticians falling foul of the rules by not checking adequately advertising copy produced on their behalf.

The GOC rescinded the rules on publicity in 2005 and no longer issue rules instead relying on the Advertising Standards Authority Codes. It should be remembered that the ASA has separate codes for broadcast and non-broadcast advertising and as the profession has developed in line with social media this should be borne in mind.

The ASA Codes are supported by sections in the GOC Standards of Practice introduced in 2010 and updated in 2020 — under Standard 16 for example it states:

> *16.4 Ensure that you do not make false or misleading statements when describing your individual knowledge, experience, expertise and specialities, including by the use of titles and*
> *16.6 Do not make misleading, confusing or unlawful statements within your advertising.*

These standards would be used should a case be brought before the fitness to practise panel.

Social media

The rapid development of social media has meant that professionals have had to be aware of the potential pitfalls of uploading information or responding to items that appear on social media. The College of Optometrists has included information on this new area of responsibility (in its published guidance 2021 Sections C134 – C153). The GOC is able to take action should posts appear that breach patient confidentiality, are inappropriate or likely to bring the profession into disrepute. In taking action the GOC will consider the legal framework, its own published standards (see Chapter 15) and guidance published by professional bodies.

As far as the GOC is concerned the following specific standards would be seen to apply to individual registrants:

- *Maintain confidentiality when communicating publicly, including speaking to or writing in the media or writing online including on social media (Standard 14 Para. 2)*
- *Ensure your conduct in the online environment, particularly regarding social media, whether or not connected to your professional practice,*

*does not damage public confidence in you or your profession
(Standard 17 Para. 3).*

The Optical Confederation has also produced "*Guidance on Social
Media and Electronic Communication*" a copy of which can be found at
https://www.fodo.com/members/guidance/category-3/social-media/. This
guidance identifies the following four areas as having the potential to
become a problem when registrants interact with social media:

- Breaches of patient confidentiality
- The blurring of professional and private boundaries
- Bringing the profession into disrepute
- Adversely impacting upon ongoing regulatory proceedings

The increasing use of electronic systems for communication and the
transfer of information make it even more important for registrants to
understand the responsibilities required when using the virtual world. The
essential message is think very carefully before uploading anything to the
virtual world.

Rules on contact lenses

Although there was only general regulation under the Opticians Act 1989
in relation to contact lenses this changed with the 2005 Amendments.
Subsequently the GOC have issued regulation and guidance on contact
lens fitting and after care by registrants. These are discussed fully in
Chapter 11.

Rules on the sale of optical appliances

Following on from the Health and Social Security Act 1984, the General
Optical Council produced the Sale of Optical Appliances Order of Council
1984 SI 1984/1778 which came into effect in December 1984. This order
deals with sale of appliances by non-qualified persons to anyone other
than:

- A person under 16 years of age.
- A person registered blind or partially sighted.

It covers the normal range of complete spectacles, frames and lenses but still does not permit the sale of contact lenses or low vision aids by the unregistered seller. Only a registered person can supply an appliance to a person under 16 years of age, and in the case of the registered sight impaired or severely sight impaired patient anything other than empty frames can only be supplied by a registered practitioner. To protect the general public SI 1984/1778 lays down certain conditions that must be fulfilled for the sale to be considered as falling within the terms of the Health and Social Security Act 1984. These conditions fall into three basic headings:

1   *Safety and serviceability conditions*
   (a) No appliance can be supplied which contains any cellulose nitrate or celluloid.
   (b) All lenses supplied had to conform to the requirements of Appendix A of BS 2738: Part 1:1989 dealing with surface defects and quality of glazing. This standard has now been replaced by BS EN ISO 21987:2017 — Ophthalmic optics — Mounted lenses.

2   *Optical performance conditions*
   In this section, the conditions are in two parts and relate either to non-complex spectacles which are defined as:

   (a) Spectacles prescribed for reading only
       with single vision spherical lenses and having a positive power not exceeding 5.00 dioptres.
   (b) Spectacles not falling within the above two categories are considered as complex spectacles (not to be confused with complex lenses).

The conditions relating to all spectacles whether they are complex or not are:

(a) The spectacles must be made according to a valid written prescription from the customer which:

(i) Has been provided by a registered medical practitioner or registered optometrist following a sight test.

(ii) Is dated not more than 2 years prior to presentation.

(b) The completed spectacles must conform to the requirements of and be within the tolerances set out in BS EN ISO 21987:2017.

3   *Additional*

Additional conditions relating to complex spectacles are as follows:

- The spectacles must be verified by focimeter as matching the written prescription.
- The spectacles must have their lenses centred according to the customer's interpupillary distance (unless otherwise specified).

If a back vertex distance is specified on the written prescription, then the supplier (or staff) must check the back vertex distance and make any allowances to the prescription that may be required to produce the necessary optical effect in the spectacles provided.

General guidelines/Standards of Practice

In the past the General Optical Council has regularly produced booklets to complement the general rules and regulations relating to optometry. These booklets contained guidance on interpretation of the rules.

Following the publication of Notice N22 in March 1987 (the updated Notice for the Guidance of the Profession) the General Optical Council decided to withdraw all guidance and to rely on rules alone. If there were any need for interpretation, then this would be left to individuals. It was decided however that where the matter related to general conduct then the Guidance of peer groups such as the British College of Optometrists would be used as it then may be taken as an indication of the professional feeling on particular matters.

In 2010 however this situation was revisited, and a new "Code of Conduct" was introduced by the GOC guiding registrants in how they were expected to behave in both their public and professional life. The

Code was replaced by the Standards of Practice in 2016 and updated in 2020. The GOC state that registrants will need to use their professional judgement in deciding how to meet the standards and to support this each element is further expanded to provide detail of expectations. These standards are used (in addition to other professional guidance) during Fitness to Practise assessments. The GOC Standards and the College of Optometrists and the GOC guidance are discussed in detail in Chapter 15.

European position

The legal situation regarding the mutual recognition of European qualifications was embodied in the general directives 89/48 EEC and 92/51 EEC for the mutual recognition of professional qualifications. Optometrists are considered under the first directive 89/48 EEC defining a general system for the recognition of higher-education diplomas awarded on completion of professional education and training of at least three years' duration. Specific recognition was included by the European Communities (Recognition of Professional Qualifications) (Amendment) Regulations 2000 (SI2000 No.1960). These were replaced subsequently by The European Communities (Recognition of Professional Qualifications) (First General System) Regulations 2005 (S.I. 2005/18). The minimum education and training period required for optometry was accepted as three year's post baccalaureate full time education leading to a university or equivalent qualification. The process for mutual recognition was provided by the EU Directive 2005/36/EC on the recognition of professional qualifications.

Provided the education and training leading to a professional qualification from a EU member state was equivalent to that in another EU member state, then the qualification was deemed as equivalent, and the holder of that qualification would not have to re-qualify and would be allowed to become a member of that profession. However, if the education and training is considerably different either in content or time then the 'host' EU member state — via the GOC in the UK — can require an aptitude test, assessments, or a period of 'supervised practice' of not more than three years without any need for re-qualifying.

Although current in 2021 there are likely to be significant changes as the political relationship between the UK and Europe changes and following the recent Education Strategic Review carried out by the GOC that resulted in changes to the expectations for provision of suitable qualification in the UK.

European Diploma in Optometry and Optics

The GOC in 2022 despite the changes to the UK's position within Europe still recognised the European Diploma in Optometry (accredited by European Council of Optometry and Optics (ECOO)) as a route to registration for non-UK applicants, however this qualification does not grant direct entry to the register and is not an Approved Qualification under the Optician's Act (Part 2 Section 8). Candidates who have passed the European Diploma in optometry will only be eligible for registration with the GOC, provided that the Council is satisfied they have demonstrated a satisfactory scope of clinical practice, and they are proficient in the English language.

Chapter 8

The Optical Services Audit
Committee and the Foresight Report

Since the Opticians Act the optical sector has produced two major reports on the provision and development of optical services. The first report was in response to political external pressures — the OSAC report — and the second in response to technological and demographic changes to population — the Foresight report.

The optometric profession throughout the 1980s came under tremendous pressure from legislative change. The Office of Fair Trading Report of 1982 seemed to release all the pressures that had been building since the Opticians Act 1958 received Parliamentary approval. Chapter 6 on the Opticians Act catalogues the changes that resulted in legislation at that time, but additional pressures arose towards the end of the 1980s.

In the build-up to the introduction of the Health and Medicines Act 1988, the Government reviewed methods of producing efficiency in the optometric services and proposed for discussion the possibility of a so-called 'two-tier' service. To some groups, the idea of a quick, inexpensive check of the refractive error with no other requirements was extremely appealing. Others concerned with the overall health care of the population found the idea an affront to the professional services that had been available for many years and that had proved so valuable to patients in health screening for both ocular and general conditions. The argument hinged on the patients' ability to decide on which 'tier' would suit their specific needs, i.e., health check or just spectacle check.

The General Optical Council took the initiative. By combining the issue of the 'two-tier' system with that of problems with unregistered sellers of spectacles and the introduction of new terms of service, the GOC proposed to the Secretary of State for Health that it should undertake a review of optical services in the UK. Upon receiving approval for the proposal, the GOC agreed on 3 July 1989 to appoint a committee to be called the Optical Services Audit Committee (OSAC). This was composed of the lay members of the General Optical Council who could be seen to have no professional or commercial conflict of interest in the services. The terms of reference given by the General Optical Council to the Committee were:

'To consider how the present and future needs of the public for the care of its vision and for the health of its eyes can best be met, by whom, and with what training and qualifications; and with what built in protection for the public, in accordance with the General Optical Council's general duty to protect the public.'

It is interesting to reflect on changes that have been introduced since the publication of the report by the Optical Services Audit Committee in 1990 and the impact it had on development of the profession in the UK.

The OSAC took information from the professional bodies concerned and all other organizations and individuals having an interest in the services and willing to take part. To assist the Committee, three specialist advisers were appointed covering the disciplines of ophthalmology, optometry, and dispensing optics.

Consultation was wide and evidence was accumulated from many different sources. In addition to meeting specific groups with a known interest and background in eye care the Committee held a public open meeting on the eye care services. Groups and individuals were invited to respond to specific questions that arose during the review and the Committee arranged to see various aspects of eye care services for itself. Eventually, one year after starting its work, the OSAC produced its report. The report had great impact on the eye care services and will be discussed as the implementation process continues today.

In the introduction the OSAC indicates that it took the objectives of the review to be as follows:

'To propose, on the basis of evidence received, a framework for optical services in the UK from 1990 onwards: and to identify those areas in which modification or development of the existing structure would be desirable for the public benefit, both in vision care and value for money in its delivery.'

The review took place against a background of legislative change, including deregulation of much of optical dispensing, including the introduction of the sale of over-the-counter reading spectacles and the abolition of the right to an NHS sight test for an estimated 60% of the population.

The report itself was divided into eight review and discussion chapters and two summary chapters. There were, in addition, several appendices giving background and detailed information for readers. The sections may for convenience be taken in terms of professional eye care, the organization and future developments of optical services, consumer interests and the European community effect.

Professional eye care

The report briefly outlined the relative roles of those responsible for eye care in the UK (ophthalmologists, ophthalmic medical practitioners, general medical practitioners, optometrists, dispensing opticians, and orthoptists) and followed this by reviewing the content of the sight test. A sight test had been taken as meaning *'a refraction and a full eye examination and such additional examinations which may be considered as clinically necessary for the patient'*, as laid down in the Sight Testing (Examination and Prescription) Regulations SI 1989/1176. This definition was in agreement with the objectives of the 'sight test' as defined by the British College of Optometrists in its guidance at the time:

- To detect ocular abnormality.
- To specify functional corrections for defects of sight.
- To suggest or provide remedial visual training where appropriate.

The review by the OSAC investigated whether there was a need to maintain the above definition and objectives or whether the public's need could be met by alternative testing methods including a direct review of the 'two-tier' proposal. This area obviously proved extremely difficult due to the many diverse arguments for retention of the status quo and as many for removal of the existing legislation, to allow anyone to provide a rapid spectacle check.

The Committee investigated self-selection of spectacles by patients, the use of auto-refractors and the possible provision by dispensing opticians of spectacle testing only. The report recommended however that the *'integrity of the sight test according to current statutory regulations should be maintained as a minimum standard in the present state of public knowledge of the sight test and eye care generally, and in the present state of visual care technology'*.

In commenting on the two-tier proposal, the OSAC did note that if public awareness were to increase to a point where informed choice by patients was possible and there were technical advances with improved performance of equipment, then a 5-year reassessment may provide a different outcome. They also noted that it might be possible to train dispensing opticians to be capable of carrying out aspects of refraction under supervision by whoever completed the eye examination and prescribed. For the objective of the OSAC to be achieved it was also recommended that both the professional bodies and the Government should carefully monitor:

- The incidence of eye disease and the numbers of sight tests performed both analysed in age groups.
- Public awareness of vision care.
- The impact of new technology on practice.

This is still ongoing despite enormous efforts by all involved and whilst there has been movement on introducing courses to enable dispensing opticians to receive exemptions for standard optometry courses and the development of specialist courses the aims have not been met. New technology has been introduced but this has had little impact on this element of eye care to date although the Foresight report predicts that this is likely to change significantly by 2030 (see later section).

Direct referral from optometrists to ophthalmologists

In reviewing the optical services, the report provided several recommendations relating to inter-professional activity. A major change to the existing procedures that the OSAC supported was the direct referral of patients to ophthalmologists when it was suspected that disease or disorder was present. To achieve this, it noted that clear criteria needed to be agreed upon between the professions and a system of notification to the general medical practitioners established. This was already starting to happen through "co-management" schemes for dealing with cataract and glaucoma referrals.

Also recommended was the monitoring of the consequences of the abolition of the NHS sight test to large numbers of the population. There were suggestions that there would be either a resultant drop in early detection of ocular disease and subsequently an increase in workload of eye departments or, alternatively, a switch of patients wanting only eye examinations to Ophthalmological departments thereby overloading the system. This was considered to be particularly important with the anticipated demographic shifts in the 1990s towards an older patient population. Early reports showed that the number of pathologies detected in the first year of the new legislation were markedly reduced and following subsequent lobbying the NHS eye examination eligibility was reinstated for the over 60-year-olds.

The Committee recommended a reversal of the overloading trend for hospital clinics and suggested that ophthalmologists, medical practitioners and optometrists discuss together ways of delegating to optometrists routine ophthalmological tasks to attempt to relieve the overload in the eye department of some NHS hospitals There was a recommendation that contractual arrangements should be made between hospitals, general medical practitioners and optometric practices and medical eye centres for the continued sight testing and monitoring of certain diseases in patients which would relieve hospital clinics of routine check-ups. It was concluded that the experience of the optometrist in the area of primary eye care would be a valuable way to relieve general medical practitioners of routine tasks relating to eye care for which they have little training.

All of these are now in place to various degrees with direct referral embedded in legislation and the development of independent prescribing by optometrists. The contracts for services rather than developing between hospital services and optometrists were driven by developments of budget shifting to Primary care Trusts and later Clinical Commissioning Groups. There is still however a long way to go and much more that could be achieved by collaborative working.

Equipment and continuing education

An area of concern to the OSAC was the standard of equipment in practice and the knowledge of new equipment. There was no specific list of equipment that should be available in a practice and indeed the British College of Optometrists when considering this found it extremely difficult to produce such a list. The College at the time had provided a breakdown of the basic eye examination requirements and indicated that suitable equipment was needed. In addition, a list of equipment was available for pre-registration supervisors to ensure adequate training opportunities.

The level of equipment in practice has steadily improved in no small measure due to competition from the influx of corporate business and patient awareness. The development of the GOS contract and practice visiting also enabled NHS England to determine that the level of equipment in practices was to a standard to meet the contract. The establishment of continuing education as a pre-condition of continued registration by the GOC also enabled training to be provided on new equipment and skills to ensure that registered practitioners kept up to date. This was of particular importance because of rapid advances in both clinical knowledge and technical optical advances.

Rationalisation

A final development in organisation foreseen by the OSAC was the rationalisation of the optical bodies and in particular the British College of

Optometrists, the Association of Optometrists, the Association of British Dispensing Opticians, the Institute of Optometry, and the British Orthoptic Society. Many of the functions undertaken by the different bodies and the training needs of their members overlapped and for efficiency and economy, and for better public awareness, it was suggested there should be a rationalisation of their functions. As would be expected with so many differing ambitions and objectives this was no easy task.

In April 2010 the Optical Confederation (OC) was launched to *"represent the 13,000 optometrists, 6,000 dispensing opticians and 7,000 optical businesses in the UK who provide high quality and accessible eye care services to the public"*. Formed as a coalition of five optical representative bodies:

- the Association of British Dispensing Opticians (ABDO);
- the Association of Contact Lens Manufacturers (ACLM);
- the Association of Optometrists(AOP);
- the Federation of Manufacturing Opticians (FMO) and
- the Federation of (Ophthalmic and Dispensing) Opticians (FODO)

this seemed to meet the aims of the OSAC report. As a Confederation they worked with others to improve eye health for the public good and the concept was that the confederation would speak with a single, authoritative voice to the Westminster government, influencers, and decision makers for the UK optical sector.

The confederation provided some notable successes for the optical sector by working together but there was still an undercurrent of self-interest for each of the bodies that surfaced from time to time and continues.

Consumer interests

The underlying theme of the OSAC report was public benefit and protection, and it was not surprising therefore that most attention had been paid to this area. The need for better promotion of information about entitlement to the NHS sight test and entitlement towards supply of spectacles following examination was expressed. It was suggested there was a need to simplify the booklet and procedures that patients were required to complete if they wished to apply for assistance towards examination and spectacle supply.

Also, it was suggested there should be a major effort to inform particular groups such as parents of young children, drivers and the visually handicapped of the range of services available and the benefits of regular examination. It was proposed that the Department of Health and the Health Education Authority, together with professional bodies, should work to achieve this end.

It is safe to say that public awareness of optical services has increased over time, but this still falls short of the ambition of the OSAC.

Optometric outlets

The downwards trend in the volume of patients attending for eye examination following removal of NHS eligibility and the rapid expansion of some optical companies provoked concern for the future of smaller independent and rural practices. It was not considered in the public interest for these to disappear and the OSAC recommended that the GOC should monitor year by year:

- The relative numbers of practices owned by corporate bodies and by independent practitioners.
- Comparative share of the market of the different types of practice.
- Comparative numbers of sight tests conducted in each.

This was in line with reservations put forward in the Crook report which formed the basic discussion document for the introduction of the 1958 Opticians Act (see Chapter 6).

The trend in volumes of patients attending for eye examination/sight testing increased over time but has plateaued recently and the larger share of the market has shifted towards the optical companies, but independent practice has held up well and some have modified their business plan shifting to offer more "niche" areas of service provision.

Consumer issues

With the specific interests of the consumer in mind the Committee reviewed the areas of contact lenses, over-the-counter reading spectacles, pricing, and prescription hand-over.

The results of their discussions and deliberations were contained in a series of recommendations. In contact lenses much had recently been achieved through the GOC contact lens registration qualification rules and it was suggested that this area should be further reviewed in the future with the intention of providing the best possible consumer service and safety at competitive costs.

The legislation allowing the purchase of ready-made reading spectacles was questioned by the OSAC based on the ability to assess needs without examination. A recommendation was made that all sales of ready-made spectacles should be accompanied by a clearly worded recommendation that the purchaser should have a sight test. The anticipated rush of patients away from practice to purchase over the counter reading spectacles has not happened and while there is a market for this route it has not significantly impacted on the eye care services.

Changes in legislation removing the NHS rights to examination and spectacles removed the previous complaint procedure that was within the control of the NHS Family Practitioner Committees. This meant that many patients were unable to follow any form of independent complaint procedure and that was obviously considered an unsatisfactory situation. A complaint procedure already existed within the profession via the Association of Optometrists who passed any complaint to the relevant organisation or individual for the most effective action, but this was not seen as independent.

The report recommended that the GOC and the professional bodies should review the situation and proposed a formal complaints procedure that would be independent, easily accessible, rapid, and able to provide binding arbitration. The method of financing of such a scheme was recognised as requiring careful consideration, particularly if the proposal to appoint an independent ombudsman was accepted. The result of this recommendation was the development of the Optical Consumer Complaints Service (OCCS) that is now well established at dealing with consumer issues (See Chapter 5). Although commissioned by the GOC and funded via registrants' fees it is a completely independent organisation.

European Community

The European Community Directive on the recognition of higher education diplomas to allow the movement of professionals throughout Europe was carefully considered. In its view, although OSAC offered no recommendations the timescale for any development was very long and it was expected that optometrists on the continent would seek to achieve the UK standard and to this end the General Optical Council would control certification and monitor UK standards.

Regulation was brought in to control movement of individuals and to assess whether qualifications obtained outside of the UK matched those required to register. In the end the GOC determines whether an applicant from outside of the UK is eligible to register to provide services and without registration it is not legal to offer the services. It will be interesting to see how the situation develops following the UKs exit from the European Union.

The Impact of the report

The report carefully studied evidence from all sectors involved with eye care, including the consumer. After weighing up all the evidence presented, the OSAC provided a series of opinions and recommendations together with a list of areas that required further consideration. While there were some sectors of the eye care service that felt disappointed at the minimal progress provided to their own aspirations, the report, as a whole, seemed to have produced well balanced conclusions. It is interesting that 30 years on it is likely that some of the same conclusions would be drawn by any committee established to carry out a similar review today. There have been changes and these have impacted on the optical sector but many of the same fundamental issues have stubbornly remained.

The Foresight Project Report

This report published in 2016 considered the potential impact of rapidly developing technology on the UK optical sector to the year 2030. Sponsored by the Optical Confederation, College of Optometrists and supported by the Central Optical Fund the report was produced by 20/20health. The aim of the report was to ensure that the optical sector was better equipped to understand as much as it could where technology, ocular medical developments and demographics were leading to in the years ahead and to inform debate as to how the optical sector could help shape and adapt to the challenges and opportunities.

The Executive Summary of the report leads with:

> *"Exponential growth of digital technology and fast-evolving demographics are altering the expectations and habits of consumers, businesses and NHS service providers. The pace of change is almost overwhelming, with automation of professional testing and measurement, DIY-health opportunities for the public, vast online resources and services, and the emancipation of research information. And yet, many of the practices and models of the optical professions have remained largely unchanged for decades."*

The report concluded that unless professionals and businesses adapt with the times, they risk becoming unviable. It was argued that in terms of technology developments in healthcare the optical sector structured as it was to rely heavily on a retail element would likely be the health sector to feel it first. It suggested that changes particularly in technology but also in an aging population and consumer attitudes meant that many medical monopolies that had enjoyed supremacy for hundreds of years had now to work out how to evolve their offering, or be dismantled from the outside in. The optical practice, in whatever form, for the future would need to give the public stronger reasons to enter its premises. This would lead to many fundamental and irreversible changes within the optical sector but at the same time produce opportunities to move forward. It was suggested that those practitioners who *"became agile, value relationships, learn how to harness the public's interest and share expertise, will be the ones who flourish"*.

The report after a general scene setting exercise is presented in 5 sections covering:

- NHS Change
- Technology and disruption
- Business impact
- Education and training
- Regulation and technology

In the context of this Chapter, it is the last section that has most relevance although it is useful to see the arguments for the likely changes to the optical sector by 2030 clearly laid out.

Below is a summary of some of the arguments included within the foresight report section on the Potential Regulatory Impact of Technology and Demographic Changes on the optical sector by 2030.

Public self-refraction

Changes to technology should enable public access to self-refraction, either as a stand-alone online service or smartphone-enabled activity. The report identifies that self-refraction is likely in at least two digital modes in the UK by 2025 and this will present significant challenges for the GOC. In addition, the report identifies that if self-refraction to produce a spectacle prescription is followed by online purchasing through overseas supply, UK regulation is fundamentally undermined and becomes toothless. Although within the UK this situation is in breach of the Opticians Act that requires a full eye health exam to be conducted by an appropriately qualified professional for a prescription to be valid, this requirement cannot be enforced outside of the UK as has been seen with attempts to enforce contact lens supply from overseas. The limiting factor for the speed of introduction and development of self-refraction will be public acceptance.

There is an additional factor here in that the NHS may decide that in the interests of public health the current system for GOS where a refraction is tied to a health check of the eyes should be retained and it is likely that a mix of financial and clinical changes may be the driver for any change. Also, the GOC by regulating the professions may make the case for consistency of care and standards and could seek to demonstrate that moving away from the current system would impact on public safety. Again, the speed of potential change is unpredictable.

Such systems are already available and the company "easee" for example claim to be the world's first CE-certified online eye exam. The test claims to be clinically validated by the Universitair Medisch Centrum Utrecht (Wisse et al 2019) but appears to be more of a screening opportunity currently. The test has however been ISO EN 13485:2016 certified by TÜV Rheinland. Several of the authors of the paper however and the funding for the validation were provided by the company and independent data are needed. The authors provide a caveat in their report:

"The Web-based tool measures the eye's visual acuity and translates this outcome into refractive error, while assuming that any error is caused solely by an uncorrected refractive error. Thus, patients with a vision-limiting eye condition, such as amblyopia, cataract, or a retinal disease, may not necessarily obtain a reliable measure of refractive error by using the Web-based tool. In practice, this effect is mitigated by including a disclaimer for patients who have such an eye condition, although the patients must be aware of having such a condition to heed this disclaimer."

This disclaimer highlights the issue of how informed patients would need to be to make an appropriate choice on their eye care as pathology is detected opportunistically during a routine sight test under current UK regulation where the patient is frequently unaware of an eye condition.

Delegated functions

Both public self-refraction and increasing in-practice automation will bring into question GOC Rules governing delegated functions. Delegated functions and supervision are discussed in more detail in Chapter 10.

The GOC's statement on the meaning of section 24 of the Opticians Act 1989 reads as follows:

"Refraction for the purpose of issuing a prescription is an essential part of the sight test. As such, refraction for the purpose of sight testing is restricted and can only be conducted by a registered optometrist, a registered medical practitioner or a student optometrist under supervision. No part of the sight test can be delegated to a dispensing optician or contact lens optician, even under supervision.

Refraction for purposes not associated with the testing of sight, for example to verify a prescription issued by an optometrist or registered medical practitioner, is not restricted. This can therefore be undertaken by dispensing opticians and contact lens opticians".

If technology, in the future, enables accurate self-refraction by members of the public how will this be reflected in the current legislation restricting the delegation of sight testing within optical practice? If the patient self-refraction were to take place within a practice setting the delegation restriction is even more directly challenged as the clinician would need to 'delegate' an important process of subjective/objective refraction to the patient. This raises the question of whether current legislation therefore implies that patient-led refraction would not be allowed in UK practice.

The current use of technician-supervised autorefraction is a delegated function of sorts, though not a full delegation since it is used only as a starting point for subjective refraction. Results from other pre-test delegated functions, for example fundus photography and visual fields require interpretation by the optometrist and their use has not been reported as presenting a direct risk to patients. If patient-led refraction were to follow this route where the optometrist validates the results obtained, then little changes in regulatory terms with the optometrist taking the responsibility.

Autorefraction: full vision testing in 2025?

Mounting pressures including from an aging population and less profitable clinical services will result in practices having to consider streamlining and automating the patient journey yet further. How then does autorefraction enabling a full vision testing fit?

The Optician's Act does not specify methods of refraction within the sight test. The Act demands such procedures as necessary 'for the purpose of detecting signs of injury, disease or abnormality in the eye or elsewhere', and states that the sight test has the objective of:

'determining whether there is any and, if so, what defect of sight and of correcting, remedying or relieving any such defect of an anatomical or physiological nature by means of an optical appliance prescribed on the basis of the determination.'

On this basis there must be some form of "sight testing" by the optometrist in order to produce a prescription, but the processes involved in how to achieve this are left to the optometrist's discretion. The lack of clarity surrounding the content of a sight test has been raised within the NHS and attempts to provide a solution over many years have not as yet been acceptable. The question then becomes whether current regulation is such that it would prevent autorefraction technology from being introduced as a standard process and it will be interesting to see what happens as technology develops more accurate systems in the future and how public expectations of their health care develop. It may be that the acceptance becomes an age-based change with younger more technologically familiar patients embracing this format but older patients more familiar with traditional care systems not wishing to change.

The offer of optometry "supervised" sight testing has already appeared in the UK during 2021 following temporary changes to regulation introduced as a result of the pandemic. To date there has been no challenge to the legality of such a service in normal circumstances. It is likely that at some point should a significant patient incident occur then the regulatory body and potentially a civil court will need to decide on whether or not this mode of practice is acceptable and meets the full regulatory framework.

The Foresight report suggests that to meet the likely future technology advances a series of questions will require consideration including:

- What are the assurances required for professionals to be able to accept and see the public as active participants in their care?
- Do we need to devise a new form of consent that allows the willing public to take more responsibility (and potentially more risk) for their health?
- What are the assurances required for regulators to be able to accept the delegation of specific responsibilities to technicians and technology?
- How can regulation enable digital technology to free up health professionals to operate to their highest capability?

The current regulation would need to be carefully reviewed and clear interpretation made to enable the potential technological led changes to be incorporated into health care as currently provided in the UK or alternatively new regulation may be required. Technological development must be seen as an opportunity and not a threat but ultimately regulation is there to ensure patient safety and consistency of care and that developments are harnessed appropriately.

The GOC in 2022 sought comment on the possibility of changing the Opticians Act to take account of some of the issues raised in the Foresight report and it will be interesting to see how this develops in the future.

Chapter 9

Continuing Education and Training/ Continuing Professional Development

Background

In 1989 the Directorate of Continuing Education and Training (DOCET) was established by the Department of Health to offer funding towards optometry training. The administration of DOCET was via the College of Optometrists and the continuing training was made available to all UK registered optometrists the only condition being that the content of the training related to the General Ophthalmic Services. This initiative led to an increase in the availability of courses. However, the DOCET funding was not extended to registered dispensing opticians.

Registered optometrists and dispensing opticians had access to continuing education lectures and courses for a considerable time before DOCET was formed but despite the introduction of DOCET there was no driver for a registrant to attend any continuing training. The situation changed when the College of Optometrists introduced a "voluntary" scheme for monitoring the uptake of Continuing Education and Training (CET) in 1995/6. This initial scheme was for College supervisors, members of College Council and members of AOP council. In 1998 the scheme was extended and made available to all UK optometry registrants. It was however still not compulsory.

During this time the GOC had reviewed its role in terms of CET and determined that a registrant should not be allowed to continue to practise without regulation to ensure updating of knowledge and skills. The GOC concluded that *"it should be a condition of retaining registration that dispensing opticians and optometrists should complete a prescribed minimum amount of CET within a stated period"* (GOC Bulletin 2004). In 2000 the Council submitted proposals for legislative change that would make this a legal requirement. The legislative processes involved however meant that it was not until 2005 and The Opticians Act 1989 (Amendment) Order (2005 SI 848) that legislation to enable the changes was finally implemented.

The GOC defined CET as the *"maintenance of up-to-date knowledge and skills required for the safe exercise of professional activities, following the obtaining of the professional qualification enabling registration"*. The GOC were careful to make the distinction between CET and Continuing Professional Development (CPD) which it considered to provide the opportunity to develop professional knowledge and skills to advance in the profession beyond the level of general registration.

The scheme

As mentioned above the scheme formally received its legal footing in 2005 with the intention of having 3-year cycles. The GOC in line with the legislation operated the first 3-year cycle from 1st January 2004 to 31st December 2006. A minimum requirement was set to achieve at least 36 "credit points" by 31st December 2006 but registrants were allowed to incorporate some points achieved via voluntary CET from 1st Jan 2004. Optometry registrants were allowed to carry forward general CET points achieved through the College voluntary scheme between the 1st January 2004 and the start date of the compulsory scheme (30th June 2005), (registered dispensing opticians were able to carry forward points from the ABDO administered voluntary scheme). Funding for managing the new scheme was proposed as being via an accreditation fee for courses, an accreditation fee for presenters and an increase in the annual levy for registrants.

It was proposed that any registrants included on a specialist list e.g., contact lens list for dispensing opticians and the yet to be introduced therapeutic supply and independent prescribing list for optometrists would be required to undertake CET specific to the specialism for retention on the list. It was anticipated that for optometrists this would be 18 "specialist" points in addition to the basic 36 points required (this was subsequently reviewed and retained). The GOC had maintained a list of all optometry registrants who had obtained, through the College voluntary scheme, a minimum of 6 points over a 3-year period to 2004. Carry over of a maximum of 6 specialist points obtained in the period 1st January 2004 to 31st December 2004 was allowed for specialist list dispensing registrants. It was also agreed that whilst not a statutory requirement the GOC would maintain a list of optometrists who after 1st January 2005 gained 6 points per year in contact lens related activity.

To ensure adequate availability of points (as all providers had to be registered and all events approved) and to fit with delivery in the existing voluntary scheme it was determined that any point achieved by approved distance learning would count in addition to any gained from attendance at approved meetings.

Under the new regulations anyone with a shortfall in points as of 1st January 2007 would be informed by the GOC and offered an opportunity to make up the points deficit by 15 March 2007. Failure to do this would mean the CET target had not been met and the name of the registrant would be removed from the register, and they would no longer be able to practise. The scheme was completely web based and it was the duty of the registrant to organise access to the web and to manage their CET points. The reason for making the scheme web based was financial as the costs for establishing and managing the scheme online were significantly lower.

In the end 90% of all registrants achieved their points requirement by 31st December 2006 the total made up of 95% optometrists, 89% dispensing opticians and 85% of contact lens specialists. This was an impressive first cycle result leading into the second cycle.

Optometry CET grants

A payment related to CET for Optometrists and OMPs in England (only) to compensate for loss of earnings in respect of undertaking continuing education and training was introduced by the Department of Health in 2004. This CET grant was taxable and not paid automatically but had to be claimed with the claimant verifying that CET had been undertaken in the previous year. The grant was not available to registered dispensing opticians but was still in place for optometrists in 2021.

The grant is paid via contractors and any optometrist that is not employed but working as a "locum" needs to make an application via one of the contractors for whom they have worked. Application is made on an annual basis for the previous year and there is a 3-month window for applications running from approximately July each year.

Amendments to the GOC scheme in 2012

The statutory requirements for the ongoing CET scheme were originally set out in *The General Optical Council (Continuing Education and Training Rules) 2005 SI1473*. There were minor amendments to the scheme once it was operating e.g., *The General Optical Council (Continuing Education and Training) (Amendment 2) Order of Council 2006 (S.I. 2006/2901)* increased the fee payable for an application to be a listed CET provider and made changes to the provisions relating to restoration and *The General Optical Council (Therapeutics and Contact Lens Specialities) Rules Order of Council 2008 (S.I. 2008/1940)* introduced a separate category of "therapeutics specialities".

Between 2009 and 2011 in response to the White Paper *'Trust Assurance and Safety'*, and the command paper *'Enabling Excellence: Autonomy and Accountability for Health and Social Care Staff'* the GOC undertook a comprehensive consultation exercise on its proposals to revalidate registrants, specifically including proposals to amend the CET scheme. The consultation exercise resulted in *The General Optical Council (Continuing Education and Training Rules) (Amendment) 2012 SI2882* introducing major changes to the CET requirements. The main purpose of the new regulations was to provide an effective and proportionate mechanism for the GOC to assure itself of registrants continued fitness to practise, to ensure that the education and training requirements were targeted to specific training needs relating to the competencies relevant to each group of professional registrants and the process for removal of a registrant from the register for failure to comply with the training requirements was robust.

The changes required a registrant to undertake education and training relevant to their scope of practise, targeted to areas of risk in optometric practise and accredited against the GOC's standards of competence and conduct relevant to each professional group. To achieve this, a registrant was required to undertake peer review events and a proportion of their CET by way of interactive methods of learning. The basis for this change was to ensure practitioners reflected on their own and others practise and did not become professionally isolated due to lack of contact with their peers. In addition, the CET undertaken by a registrant had to demonstrate up to date knowledge and skill across all the GOC's standards of competence and conduct relevant for their professional group and scope of practise. This development meant that a registrant could not just pick a single area of practise in which to achieve the required CET points.

Removal from the register

The process for removal of a registrant's name for failure to meet the CET requirements also was amended. The existing scheme allowed for a three-month period at the end of the cycle to enable a registrant to make up any shortfall of training points. However, it was identified that some registrants treated the shortfall period as an extended period of the cycle in which to complete their cycle of training. The changes removed the shortfall period so that a registrant no longer had the additional period between 1st January and 1st April to make up any shortfall before a decision to remove their name from the register was made by the registrar. This was intended to maximise the protection of the public by ensuring that those who had not undertaken the required training were removed from the register as soon as possible at the end of the three-year cycle. As a safeguard for registrants the changes included that notice should be given to registrants who had not met the requirements two months before the end of the three-year cycle warning them that if they failed to achieve the requirements by the end of the cycle, they may be removed from the register from the 1st January.

The decision to remove a registrant from the register may be appealed under the Opticians Act 1989. The registrant can appeal to the Registration Appeals Committee within 28 days of the decision being made. The decision to remove is suspended for those 28 days and if an appeal is lodged within that time is further suspended until the Committee makes a final decision and the registrant may make up any shortfall in requirements during this period.

Specialities

The final amendment was to simplify aspects relating to specialities. The specialities open to registrants are set out in the General Optical Council (Registration Rules) 2005 SI1478. A dispensing optician may have the contact lens specialty and an optometrist may have one or more of the therapeutics specialties. The requirement is that only one set of specialty points needs to be undertaken regardless of whether this is a contact lens speciality or one or more therapeutics specialty.

The GOC developed an IT system to support the scheme providing a web-based repository for every registrant CET portfolio. The system supported auditing of 100% of registrant portfolios on a three-yearly basis to determine compliance with the requirements and annual monitoring to track those not on target. Additional sampling and targeted auditing of portfolios via the web-based CET platform enabled assessment of the quality of registrant reflection statements and portfolios. A registrant was able to view their own details at any time.

CET approval

All CET provision required advance approval using a process of assessment against the GOC standards of competence and conduct, this provided assurance as to the relevance and suitability of CET. Feedback by registrants was recorded on the system and used to support the evaluation of the effectiveness of the scheme and of individual providers of CET. As part of the quality control process all providers initially had to submit proposed courses for approval although over time some large providers were able to operate a slightly different system.

A new scheme for 2022

In 2016/17 the GOC determined the need to review its education strategy for both undergraduate, pre-reg and ongoing professional development and began a public consultation. Over the next 4 years the whole system was reviewed as part of the GOC "Education Strategic Review", and new processes and requirements put in place. The main aim of the review was to ensure that education programmes and qualifications leading to GOC registration equipped students to meet patients' future needs, as technological change and the increased prevalence of enhanced services were altering the roles that optometrists and dispensing opticians played in delivering eye care. It was felt that the optical sector was undergoing major change and forward thinking was required as optical professionals would need to be fully equipped to tackle the challenges of the coming decades, working closely with other professionals as part of a flexible healthcare workforce.

The current system for CPD was developed following the extensive consultation undertaken as part of the Education Strategic Review and introduced in 2022. It was concluded that there was a need to change the requirements for CET for all registrants. The GOC found that there was significant support for evolving the existing scheme and

- Replacing the competencies — these were seen as overly prescriptive
- Allowing registrants more control over their learning and development and the ability to tailor it to their own personal scope of practice
- Enhancing requirements for registrants to reflect on their practice
- Changing the name of the scheme from CET to Continuing Professional Development (CPD).
- Introducing a new proportionate system of CPD approvals

CET to CPD

The re-brand of the CET scheme to CPD had been well supported and was introduced at the start of the new 3-year cycle in January 2022. It was felt that the name of the scheme should reflect the other changes made from

2022. The requirements moved the new scheme away from appearing to maintain core competencies towards promoting lifelong learning and development throughout a registrant's professional career. The change in name also provided consistency with the approach taken by other healthcare regulators and minimised the risk of the GOC scheme being perceived as an inferior scheme.

Standards of Competence to Standards of Practice for Registrants

The new CPD scheme from 1st January 2022 moved from using the GOC standards of competence for education as the underpinning driver to using the *"Standards of Practice for Optometrists and Dispensing Opticians"*. Using the standards of competence for education to underpin the scheme had given the impression that it was a maintenance scheme to keep registrants at the level they were at when they graduated and not for development. It was felt that there was a need to offer registrants more control over their learning and development and this required a move away from the rigid and overly prescriptive format to encourage and facilitate genuine learning and development for registrants.

The Standards of Practice for Optometrists and Dispensing Opticians cover the wide set of professional skills and responsibilities required of all individual GOC registrants and are considered to be a more appropriate underpin for a scheme focused on professional development.

The key components of the scheme were illustrated in the GOC consultation document in 2021 and demonstrated a mix of the existing scheme and the new scheme (see Fig. 1). The Standards of Practice underpinning the new CPD scheme were grouped within four domains and a registrant is required to achieve at least one piece of CPD in each of the four main domains during the 3-year cycle. This applies to all registrants, including those who are also contact lens opticians (CLOs) or therapeutic prescribers (TPs). A new mandatory reflective learning exercise was introduced to be undertaken during a 3-year cycle.

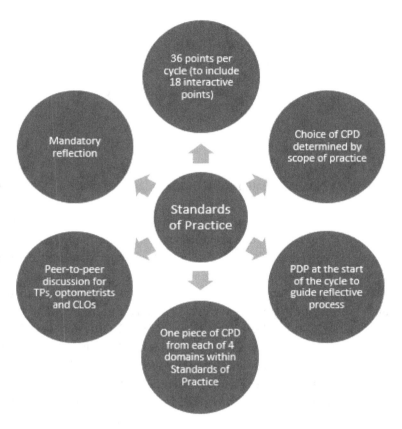

Figure 1:   Overview of key components of the CPD scheme (Reproduced with kind permission of the GOC from CPD (CET) review proposals consultation — final report GOC Sept. 2020)

It was not all change however and the requirement to obtain 36 points over a three-year cycle, of which a minimum of 18 must be interactive CPD was retained, optometrists with specialist listing as TPs still must obtain an additional 18 points in their specialty meaning 54 points in total (CLOs must complete 18 of their 36 points in their specialty). Registrants are required to plan their CPD for the three-year cycle and Optometrists, TPs and CLOs must undertake at least one peer-to-peer discussion per 3-year cycle.

Table 1:   The Four Domains for CPD

Domain 1: Professionalism
Domain 2: Communication
Domain 3: Clinical practice
Domain 4: Leadership and accountability

Domains

The four new domains created from the Standards of practice are shown in Table 1.

In addition to these four main domains two additional "Areas" were introduced — Area A covers specialty requirements and Area B was designed to enable the GOC to rapidly address any identified risks by requiring specific training. Existing requirements for contact lens opticians and therapeutic prescribers to undertake CPD in relation to their specialty fell within Area A. However, Area B was more flexible and provided the GOC with the option to set targeted CPD for a cycle and specify who undertook this CPD in areas related to risk, for example, newly qualified registrants could be required to undertake CPD targeted at their transition into clinical practice (instead of CPD in the four main domains). It was also seen as a way of addressing or filling known gaps in skill sets or dealing with any issues that may be raised through the FTP process that affected all registrants.

Table 2 indicates how the GOC Standards of Practice correspond with the four CPD domains.

Non-approved CPD

In the scheme prior to 2022 all CET went through an approval process before it could be offered to a registrant, this took no account of CPD undertaken with other professionals or for example as part of a contract with the NHS. The GOC considered this interprofessional learning extremely valuable and essential for the development of the optical professions.

From 1st January 2022 a registrant was allowed to achieve points when participating in CPD that had not been formally approved for the

Table 2: **Standards of Practice and Domains** (Reproduced with kind permission of the GOC from CPD A guide for registrants (2021))

Domain 1: Professionalism
- *Show care and compassion for your patients (s.4)*
- *Work collaboratively with colleagues in the interests of patients (s.10)*
- *Protect and safeguard patients, colleagues and others from harm (s.11)*
- *Show respect and fairness to others and do not discriminate (s.13)*
- *Maintain confidentiality and respect your patients' privacy (s.14)*
- *Maintain appropriate boundaries with others (s.15) Be honest and trustworthy (s.16)*
- *Do not damage the reputation of your profession through your conduct (s.17)*
- *Be candid when things have gone wrong (s.19)*

Domain 2: Communication
- *Listen to patients and ensure they are at the heart of decisions made about their care (s.1)*
- *Communicate effectively with patients (s.2)*
- *Obtain valid consent (s.3)*
- *Respond to complaints effectively (s.18)*

Domain 3: Clinical practice
- *Keep your knowledge and skills up to date (s.5)*
- *Recognise, and work within, your limits of competence (s.6)*
- *Conduct appropriate assessments, examinations, treatments and referrals (s.7)*

Domain 4: Leadership and accountability
- *Maintain adequate patient records (s.8)*
- *Ensure that supervision is undertaken appropriately and complies with the law (s.9)*
- *Ensure a safe environment for your patients (s.12)*

purposes of the GOC CPD scheme. This self-directed CPD allows a registrant to count learning from wider sources towards their points total and provides an opportunity to include relevant learning with others outside of the sector. There is no requirement for a registrant to include this form of learning and it will not necessarily be suitable for all registrants.

Self-directed learning has been defined by Moja et al. 2015 as *"an active learning approach in which learners take autonomy over the learning process, selecting what to learn, how to learn it, and where and when to engage in the learning."*

For a GOC registrant to include such learning it must meet certain criteria:

- it is at least one hour long;
- it has been developed for professionals involved in healthcare;
- a written statement was made after completing the CPD to explain why it was relevant to a registrant's own CPD; and
- no more than 50% of a registrant's overall total CPD came from non-approved CPD sources.

This means that a minimum of 50% of a registrant's CPD must come from approved CPD sources. All non-approved CPD gains a standard one point for every hour undertaken up to a maximum of three points per activity. To ensure quality and to prevent any abuse of the system the GOC introduced an audit system whereby 10% of registrants completing non-approved CPD are audited each year.

Reflective learning statements

Reflection had become an increasingly important part of CPD schemes as a mechanism for embedding good practice and improving patient care. The GOC as part of the CET/CPD reforms enhanced requirements for registrants to reflect on their practice and ensured this became a core part of the new scheme. When making this decision the GOC identified the following potential barriers to reflection

- lack of clarity around/understanding of the concept and benefits of reflective practice;
- a fear of reprisal for being open and honest about where mistakes have been made or where things could have been done better;
- the perception that reflective practice was simply a box-ticking exercise; and
- a lack of guidance and support to enable registrants to reflect effectively.

There were however many registrants under the old scheme who were effectively using reflection and the GOC to build on this and to break down the barriers issued new guidance to all registrants to cover the above issues.

Registrants are still required to plan their CPD at the start of each cycle and optometrists and CLOs must complete at least one peer-to-peer discussion in a three-year cycle and reflect upon the session.

Registrants are also advised to complete a short, written reflection after any CPD activity as this informs the newly introduced requirement for all registrants to carry out and document, with a peer, a reflective exercise about their CPD plan, what has been undertaken and broader professional development either during or at the end of a 3-year cycle. This new requirement was considered important as having given registrants more control over the CPD they select the GOC needed assurance that registrants were reflecting on their practice and had tailored their CPD to their own learning and development needs.

Table 3 sets out the elements of reflection expected by the GOC at various points in the 3-year cycle.

The GOC consider that a peer could be another registrant, an employer or a statutorily regulated healthcare professional from a different discipline but could not be a relative, close friend or employee. Registrants are asked to self-declare that their CPD Plan/other planning documents have been completed and self-declare the discussion has been completed. The peer must sign the registrant's written reflection to confirm the

Table 3: Elements of reflection for CPD (Reproduced with kind permission of the GOC from CPD (CET) review proposals consultation — final report GOC Sept. 2020)

Start of CPD cycle	*1. CPD Planning*
	2. New GOC guidance on reflection issued
During CPD Cycle	*1. Peer-to-peer discussion undertaken by optometrists and CLOs*
	2. Optional additional reflection after each activity
	3. All registrants to complete mandatory reflective exercise on their CPD plan with a peer or other healthcare professional (alternatively this can be done at the end of the cycle)
End of CPD Cycle	*All registrants to complete mandatory reflective exercise on their CPD plan with a peer or other healthcare professional (if not already done so)*

peer-reflection has been undertaken. To ensure compliance the GOC randomly audit a selection.

CPD approvals

Prior to 2022 all applications for CET activities had to be approved in advance of the activity being delivered to registrants (referred to as 'up-front approvals'). This process was costly and time-consuming both for the GOC and the provider. As part of the GOC's review it was decided that a lighter touch was required but that quality assurance processes were still necessary to ensure quality of future provision. The result was a shift to a more proportionate approach approving and auditing CPD providers rather than approving individual events and sessions. Approved providers were still to be registered and required to demonstrate understanding of the requirements of CPD delivery and the capability to deliver CPD to a high standard. A provider audit scheme would undertake an annual review, and this was established to:

- Benchmark the standards expected of CPD providers
- Provide a paper-based audit of providers taking account of registrant feedback and complaints to identify any that may be considered 'at risk'
- Undertake targeted auditing of providers identified as 'at risk'
- Carry out a general audit of 10% of all registered providers each year.

It is anticipated that the new scheme will create greater flexibility and interest for participants and promote greater acceptance of CPD.

Chapter 10

Delegation and Supervision

Several cases have appeared before GOC Fitness to Practise panels related to the processes of delegated function and of supervision. It is acceptable for certain test procedures within the eye examination to be delegated providing the person carrying out the function has been trained and is being supervised. In addition, there are several situations within optometry where other forms of supervision are required not least in the case of mentoring a pre-registration student. It is important therefore to know the regulatory structure for such activities. This is becoming even more important with the potential developments outlined in the Foresight report (See Chapter 8).

What is delegation?

The dictionary definition of delegation is '*entrusting a task to another*' (Pocket Oxford Dictionary 1992). There doesn't seem to be a legal definition for delegation in a clinical setting relating to optical functions in the UK. There are definitions in other disciplines in other countries. The College of Physicians and Surgeons of Nova Scotia for example published in 2005 the following for delegated medical functions that in general terms may be considered appropriate:

> "A ***delegated medical function*** (DMF) *is a procedure/ treatment/intervention that falls within the practice of medicine ..... that in the interests*

of client/patient care, has been approved by the regulatory bodies of both medicine and nursing to be performed by registered nurses with the required competence (i.e., certification)."

In UK Optics there has been no approval from the regulatory body (General Optical Council) on the clinical functions that could be delegated or what level of training/accreditation/supervision would be acceptable to enable someone to carry out delegated functions. The Opticians Act 1989 does however restrict the testing of sight to registered optometrists and certain other professional groups but does not specify which tests are restricted. Anecdotally within UK optics a delegated function has been seen as one that an individual undertakes at the request of a clinician that provides clinical data for the clinician to then interpret. The GOC recently issued a statement of clarification referring to a case in which it had been suggested at a Fitness to Practise hearing that refraction under supervision by a dispensing optician was an accepted delegated function within a sight test. The GOC statement reads:

"Refraction for the purpose of issuing a prescription is an essential part of the sight test. As such, refraction for the purpose of sight testing is restricted and can only be conducted by a registered optometrist, a registered medical practitioner or a student optometrist under supervision. No part of the sight test can be delegated to a dispensing optician or contact lens optician, even under supervision.

Refraction for purposes not associated with the testing of sight, for example to verify a prescription issued by an optometrist or registered medical practitioner, is not restricted. This can therefore be undertaken by dispensing opticians and contact lens opticians."

In 2022 the GOC were seeking opinion on whether this was still a sensible approach or should be modified.

Why delegate?

In optical practice the main reason for delegation is efficiency. Optometrists are the most expensive commodity in a practice and delegating specific tasks that involve a machine that measures data to a lower cost member of staff releases the optometrist's time to see more patients and leads to increased patient throughput and ultimately increased efficiency/profitability without risk to patients. The same reasoning can be applied to the delegation of teaching the insertion and removal of contact lenses by a contact lens optician, another expensive commodity in a practice setting.

Who can carry out delegated functions?

As mentioned above there appear to be no regulations within UK optics specifying who is able to carry out a delegated function. The College of Optometrists however has issued guidance (updated 2021) on this area that is consistent with guidance from other professional bodies. When an optometrist delegates a function, according to College guidance:

> *"The optometrist has a duty to ensure that the patient receives the same standard of care whether or not s/he delegates any task and to satisfy him/herself as to the competence and suitability of the person to perform the task being delegated".*

This means that only individuals who have received appropriate training and shown themselves to be competent and suitable for the delegated task should be undertaking such tasks. Should a complaint arise that involves a delegated task the delegating optometrist takes responsibility. It would be for the optometrist to prove that the individual to whom a task had been delegated was indeed competent and suitable and that a patient did not receive a lower standard of care. Ultimately patient safety would be the deciding factor.

A paper by Bosley and Dale looked at the use of Health Care Assistants (HCAs) to whom tasks could be delegated in Hospital and General Medical Practice and the authors noted that there was very little literature on the topic and wrote:

> *"The key to promoting patient safety is to ensure that HCAs are trained and competent to undertake the tasks delegated to them, and that accountability is clear.... Practice nurses are commonly responsible for delegating to HCAs, and accountable for the appropriateness of delegation. To make such decisions appropriately, they need to ensure that*

HCAs have the knowledge, skills, and competence to undertake the delegated tasks, taking into account the individual's own confidence and experience. The RCN advises that HCAs should work according to defined protocols and procedures, and that they should not be asked to make clinical judgements. HCAs should be accountable to a registered healthcare professional and receive regular supervision..... If the legal parameters of the role are unclear to staff who are delegating work, HCAs' skills may be under-utilised or, conversely, they may be asked to work beyond their capabilities. Research suggests that in the pressured hospital environment, the latter is sometimes the case. Busy staff in general practice also experience the conflicting demands of immediate patient need and remaining within the parameters of safety.'" (Bosley and Dale 2008)

In an optical practice delegated tasks are performed by a wide variety of staff with a range of training, qualifications, and competencies. Due to the structures within optical practices and lack of agreed clarity, functions have often been delegated by default to a non-qualified member of staff with a minimum of training, no formal assessment and working to unclear legal parameters which, as noted in the above paper, may lead to underutilisation of skills or people being asked to work beyond their capabilities. It would be very useful therefore to have clear agreed boundaries in optics to help ensure patient safety alongside efficiency. It is important however to reiterate that no-one should be performing a task on a patient unless suitably trained and accredited and under adequate supervision and that it is the responsibility of the person delegating to ensure that 'assistants' have the appropriate knowledge and skills to ensure patient safety.

Who delegates?

Within optical practice there is opportunity for optometrists, dispensing opticians, and contact lens opticians to delegate specific tasks. As mentioned above these are tasks that the individual to whom they are delegated would carry out under supervision with the person delegating retaining responsibility for patient care at all times. Examples of functions currently being delegated are shown in table 1.

Table 1:   Examples of delegated functions

Optometrists
- Non-contact Tonometry
- Digital imaging/OCT
- Visual Field screening
- Auto refraction

Optometrists and Dispensing Opticians
- Frame measurement
- Lens centres and heights
- Frame adjustment
- Repairs

Optometrists and Contact lens opticians
- Insertion and removal teaching
- Keratometry

What cannot be delegated?

As mentioned above Statutory functions relating to the testing of sight and contact lens fitting as laid out in the Opticians Act 1989 sections 25 and 26 and Sight Testing (Examination and Prescription) (No2) Regulations 1989 cannot be delegated. The College of Optometrists guidance states: '*Optometrists are reminded that the protected functions of sight testing and contact lens fitting cannot be delegated. This would include any part of the sight testing or contact lens fitting that would be regarded as assessing the patient or exercising clinical judgement*'

This raises a further consideration — the blurring of margins around delegated functions i.e., whether measuring or interpretation or both are statutory functions. For example, in the case of field plots — is carrying out an automated field test a statutory function when a 'clinical' assessment of a patient's speed of response or lack of concentration during a test may be an essential factor in assessing the outcome or does interpreting a field plot printed following testing by a non-registered assistant fulfil the statutory function? In contact lens fitting is inserting a lens for the purpose of assessing fit a statutory function or is it the assessment of the fit of a lens initially inserted by a non-registered assistant that it the statutory function?

Without clear legal parameters or at least widely accepted custom and practice it is not possible to answer these questions consistently. Within optics it is likely that different professionals looking at delegation would have different views.

In some cases, it isn't just the task being delegated but the content of the task that raises an issue. For example, non-contact tonometry to measure intra ocular pressure may be considered an acceptable delegated function but contact tonometry requiring anaesthesia and touching the eye surface with a potentially higher risk to the patient may not be considered acceptable for delegation.

There is also a question mark over the legality of an assistant who has completed a measurement of the visual field or a non-contact tonometry saying to the patient "That result is normal" when the field plot or intra-ocular pressures results have not been assessed by a registered clinician and placed within the context of other findings. This is effectively making a clinical judgement that the individual is not qualified to make.

It could be suggested therefore that a screening task that automatically records data does not form part of the sight test (such as non-contact tonometry) and may be acceptable for delegation whereas the measurement of visual fields may or may not depending on one's viewpoint. However, should the visual fields or tonometry be abnormal or the result form part of the clinical decision-making process of a sight test they may need to be repeated personally by the optometrist/clinician to be valid.

Delegation and dispensing of spectacles

The deregulation of the sale and supply of spectacles by the Sale of Optical Appliances Order 1984 resulted in an opportunity for the sale and supply of spectacles in an optical practice to be undertaken by non-registered employees. Exceptions to this form of supply which still fall within the terms of section 27(1) of the Opticians Act 1989 are spectacles supplied to persons under 16 years of age and persons registered as blind or partially sighted where any sale must be affected by or under the supervision of a registered dispensing optician, registered optometrist, or registered medical practitioner.

The GOC has heard Fitness to Practise cases relating to non-supervision of a sale to a patient under 16 years of age. Outcomes from Fitness to Practise panel decisions have reiterated that there is a need for supervision to be by a registered optometrist or dispensing optician who must be on the premises and in a position to intervene. The need for supervisory duties to be established by written contract to ensure clarity for all concerned also has been stressed.

Supervision

The legal definition of supervision has generally been taken as that given in a High Court judgement relating to supply of a pharmaceutical product. In the judgement in *Roberts v Littlewoods Mail Order Stores Ltd (1943)* it was shown that a sale of a restricted item was made while the pharmacist was in a stockroom upstairs and unaware of the transaction by an unqualified assistant. It was held by the High Court that supervision had not been present and in summing up the case Lord Caldicott recorded that:

> *"It has been suggested that a man can supervise a sale without being bodily present. I do not accept that contention ... each individual sale must be not necessarily effected by the qualified person but something which is shown by the evidence to be under his supervision in the sense that he must be aware of what is going on at the counter and in a position to supervise or superintend the activities of the young woman by whom each individual sale is effected."*

The General Optical Council has issued a statement outlining the requirements for those supervising trainees or those undertaking delegated activities that would demonstrate to the GOC that the supervision is *adequate*.

The definition is that 'adequate supervision' is provided by a registrant who:

- is sufficiently qualified and experienced to themselves undertake the functions they are supervising;

- is not only on the premises but in a position to oversee the work undertaken and to intervene if necessary, in order to ensure protection of the patient;
- retains clinical responsibility for the patient;
- ensures that no untoward consequences to the detriment of the patient can arise from the actions of a person who is being supervised;
- ensures compliance with all legal requirements governing the activity.

Where the supervision relates to trainees undertaking practice-based learning this must take place under the supervision of an appropriately qualified, registered, and approved supervisor. To supervise in this situation, the supervisor must:

- *Have at least two years recent and relevant post qualification practical experience;*
- *Have maintained a minimum of two years continuous GOC registration;*
- *Comply with the GOC code of conduct in their professional practice;*
- *Ensure that your students are registered with the GOC;*
- *Meet the approval criteria of Providers;*
- *Provide continuous personal supervision, i.e., be in the practice when the student is in professional contact with patients and be able to intervene as necessary;*
- *Support, observe and mentor;*
- *Provide a sufficient and suitable learning environment;*
- *Ensure the student has access to the appropriate equipment to meet the requirements of the Route to Registration;*
- *Be familiar with the assessment requirements, guidelines, and regulations of the Route to Registration;*
- *Ensure that when the student is in professional contact with patients they are clearly identified as a trainee under supervision and that the identity of the supervisor is also made clear to the patient.*

This is consistent with the use of the basic term supervision in the College of Optometrists guidance:

"The supervisor must be on the premises, aware of the procedure and in a position to intervene if necessary to ensure that no untoward consequences to the detriment of the patient can arise from the actions of such a person who is being supervised".

The requirements of supervision were further explored by the case of *General Optical Council v Vision Direct (1989)*. In this case held before magistrates it was held that supervision by an optometrist (or dispensing optician) means that the optometrist (or dispensing optician) when supervising is able to exercise his or her professional skill and judgement as a clinician. It does not mean supervision by someone performing a purely clerical or even management function, even if the person who is performing that function happens to be a registered optometrist (or dispensing optician).

All delegated functions should be carried out only when the person delegating and taking responsibility is on the premises to provide supervision.

Further support for this view of supervision can be found in two Clinical Governance toolkits (England and Wales) developed jointly by the optical organizations (AOP, FODO, ABDO and the College of Optometrists). The optical bodies believe these should become models for clinical governance in England and Wales.

When discussing supervision one of the core standards in the toolkit is: *"clinical care and treatments are carried out under appropriate clinical supervision and leadership."*

As a way of achieving this it is noted that: *"Where tasks within the sight test, or dispensing to restricted groups, are delegated to others, practitioners must ensure that those undertaking the delegated tasks are appropriate and suitably trained. At all times a supervising optometrist or dispensing optician (as appropriate) must be present in the practice. Guidance as to who can or cannot carry out specific delegated tasks, and under what circumstances, should be available in writing within the practice."* Whilst this offers a degree of ambiguity by not defining what are the statutory functions of the sight test that cannot be delegated or the training requirements, it does attempt to identify boundaries.

It identifies that it is essential that standard operating procedures are in place for all delegated tasks and that the individual supervising and the individual being supervised are clear on the roles and boundaries for the tasks. It is also important according to the GOC code for business registrants to take reasonable and proportionate steps to *"not knowingly act in a way which might contribute to or cause a breach of the Code of Conduct for Individual Registrants by any individual registrant employed or otherwise engaged by it to provide optical services"* and *"to ensure that each person who undertakes activities regulated by the Opticians Act does so in accordance with the Act."*

General direction and direction

A further aspect of supervision relates to 'general direction' and 'direction'. The Opticians Act 27(3)(d) states that contact lenses may be sold by a person *'if the seller is, or is under the general direction of, a registered medical practitioner, a registered optometrist or a registered dispensing optician'*.

If the sale is made under the general direction of an optometrist, the law requires that the seller verify the particulars of the specification with the person who issues it. Guidance from the College of Optometrists are consistent on general direction and require that:

> *"where the supply of lenses is under the general direction of a registered optometrist/dispensing optician, the generally directing individual should ensure that robust procedures are in place to protect the patient. A generally directing optometrist/dispensing optician has a responsibility to ensure that the systems used for verification and supply are robust and are followed. Whilst the generally directing optometrist/dispensing optician need not be on the premises while the sale takes place, any protocol for such supply should be in writing with an audit trail that can be followed. The protocol should include the requirement for suppliers to be adequately trained and to have working knowledge of the types of contact lenses available and the different care regimes. Suppliers should be trained to advise the patient appropriately as to what to do if the patient suffers an adverse event from the use of the lenses or care solutions."*

There is an additional note however that suppliers working under general direction should *"not interpret or make judgements in relation to any clinical information contained in the specification, and should refer such matters to an optometrist, dispensing optician or registered medical practitioner and seek direction from them."*

This identifies a difference between general direction, which is overseeing a process, and direction which relates to a specific individual clinical action. The requirements under direction are therefore more onerous than those under general direction. Direction also comes into play for example with the instillation of Tropicamide where the task has been delegated. According to the College of Optometrists *"The use of pupil dilating eye drops should always be done under the direction and supervision of an optometrist"* requiring both clinical direction for an individual patient and supervision of the task. The important issue here is that only the optometrist (or OMP) is entitled to be supplied with Tropicamide and use the drug in a practice and therefore if the drug is given by an optometrist for instillation by a non-clinician who would be unable to legally obtain the drug for use by themselves the optometrist remains responsible for its use.

Section 9 of the GOC Standards of Practice for optometrists covers supervision and delegation. It makes it clear that the GOC's view is that supervision should not compromise patient care and safety and that both the supervisor and those being supervised share a responsibility for the patient. According to the Guidance adequate supervision requires a clinician to:

- Be sufficiently qualified and experienced to undertake the functions being supervising.
- Only delegate to those who have appropriate qualifications, knowledge, or skills to perform the delegated activity.
- Be on the premises, in a position to oversee the work undertaken and ready to intervene if necessary, in order to protect patients.
- Retain clinical responsibility for the patient. When delegating responsibility is retained for the delegated task and for ensuring that it has been performed to the appropriate standard.
- Take all reasonable steps to prevent harm to patients arising from the actions of those being supervised.

- Comply with all legal requirements governing the activity.
- Ensure that details of those being supervised or performing delegated activities are recorded on the patient record.

Patient safety

Whatever the process of delegation the ultimate goal as shown by the GOC standard is to maintain patient safety — it would be totally inappropriate and unacceptable to put a patient at risk through a task being delegated. The regulation and guidance from many professional bodies relating to clinical delegation appear to include training, competency, clarity of role and setting of boundaries as means of ensuring patient safety

Standards of training and accreditation

There are several academic institutions offering training and a qualification to dispensing opticians and optical assistants that includes elements of delegated functions. However as has been discussed there is little regulatory framework to inform course content which is based around current practice. Many optical companies provide in house training for qualified and non-qualified staff but much of the practical training for delegated tasks is carried out at practice level. Training is often either by a resident optometrist or by a non-qualified assistant who has been carrying out the task but may have no skill in training or may not have been assessed themselves to ensure they are performing the task adequately. This is likely to lead to poor consistency. In independent practice an optometrist may take the time to train an assistant to reach a standard with which they are comfortable, but comfort zones may differ between practitioners.

The question becomes how much is passed on during training to enable a task to be completed to the same level as the person delegating? The example raised earlier related to how many clinical assistants carrying out a field check are aware of the potential clinical importance of observed patient performance problems or consider passing these on if noticed.

There would be sense in reviewing the whole area of training and assessment in relation to delegation to ensure that patient safety is not put at risk by inadequate or inappropriate training. This would require the establishment of a system of transportable accreditation of competency to provide consistency that was recognised across optics.

Responsibility

It seems to be generally accepted that in a clinical situation the person delegating retains responsibility for the patient care and outcomes. It is also clear from literature and guidance that the person to whom tasks are delegated should be competent and suitable to perform the tasks. As stated above however this is very difficult to confirm — without formal accreditation or direct monitoring of individuals it is not possible to know the standard to which they work. A new non-clinical staff member coming from another practice may say that they routinely carry out field tests but to what standard?

This level of acceptance of responsibility is more difficult for a locum optometrist who still is required to ensure, if delegating, that they are satisfied that the individual to whom a task is delegated is competent and suitable. The question arises as to how this is possible? Moving between practices unless there is a system of training and assessing at each practice attended it would be impossible to guarantee the standard of an individual. Do all practices have training programmes? Are all training programmes equivalent? Does receiving training provide evidence of competency or knowledge or both? A contractor's assurance that a non-qualified staff member is able to perform a task to an acceptable standard may not be a satisfactory defence for a delegating optometrist if the staff member is shown later not to be competent.

Decision making

It is important to remember that when delegating, an optometrist, according to the College of Optometrists guidance:

> *"makes all decisions with regard to the patient's clinical care and at all times retains responsibility for the patient, for the work of the person to*

whom tasks are delegated and for the outcome of the examination findings".

The College guidelines state that *"non optometrists to whom tasks are delegated should not be expected or asked to interpret any findings that may be obtained by them in the course of carrying out those tasks"*. This would mean that the person to whom field screening is delegated is not able to make the decision that the plot is normal. The delegating optometrist should check every plot (and preferably sign it off) to ensure that someone else does not make the clinical decision. Non- registered staff should be aware that they should not be advising patients on the potential outcome of clinical tasks they have had delegated to them even by saying the results are normal.

Insurance

At present there is no specific insurance available for individuals carrying out a delegated function, as stated earlier individuals carrying out delegated tasks do so under supervision. The insurance of the individual delegating should cover the task although this may be questioned if the delegation falls outside the legal framework. This puts an onus on the individuals with insurance to be aware of what is happening in their name and to ensure that their insurance covers them for the task being delegated. It also puts an onus on an employer to ensure that insurance is in place to cover all eventualities for the services they are providing. (See Chapter 17)

Are these issues only relevant to optics?

All professions as they progress have decisions to make on roles and functions. The pharmacy profession reviewed its own guidance in the light of the Medicines Act 2006 that established enabling legislation that would allow wider delegation within pharmacy services although supervision is still strict in terms of what may be delegated and to whom. It paved the way for accredited and registered pharmacy technicians to play an increasing role in the supply process. During the consultation phase the Royal Pharmaceutical Society in its response had to consider how such a process may work to maintain patient safety and professional responsibility while still opening up supply. The final outcome may impact on other professions.

The medical and nursing professions have been looking at delegation and supervision for some time. The following passage is taken from a paper published in 2004 looking at the role of Health Care Assistants in Nursing: *"While they represent a substantial proportion of the health care workforce, the growth of their role has taken place without regulation, clear boundaries, or systematic education and training. This has raised serious concerns, especially with regard to the issues of patient safety and quality of care. For health professionals, regulations, role clarity and validated education and training are key elements of ensuring the safety of the public"*. (McKenna HP, Hasson F, Keeney S 2004).

It is time for the optical profession to revisit supervision and delegation and whether it should be allowed to evolve unchecked or whether there should be some ground rules as to what is acceptable in line with those in other professions. The GOC as part of its review of the Opticians Act in 2022 asked for comments on delegation of elements of the sight test and it will be interesting to see the outcome of this.

Chapter 11

Rules and Guidance Relating to Contact Lenses

Prior to June 1985, the General Optical Council had no published rules on the fitting and supply of contact lenses. The Council had, however, issued guidance on these matters which had been regularly updated and which before the introduction of the 1985 rules fell within the simple statement:

'In order to protect both individual patients and the public at large, it must be made clear that in relation to all registered opticians' professional activities, it is beholden upon the individual to maintain the highest standards of experience, training, performance and behaviour.'

Many practitioners felt that this was inadequate and the General Optical Council itself drew up draft regulations for contact lens practice which were initially rejected by the Privy Council on the grounds that the proposed rules were outside the scope of the legal duty of the General Optical Council.

Under the terms of the Opticians Act 1958, the General Optical Council was given permission to make rules prohibiting or regulating the prescription, supply, and fitting of contact lenses by registered opticians, enrolled bodies corporate, and their employees, but not covering subsequent follow-up of the patient.

Who can fit Contact Lenses?

The Health and Social Security Act 1984 introduced a new section to the Opticians Act 1958, to deal with certain aspects of contact lens work. This was changed by s. 25 of the Opticians Act 1989, which restricts the fitting of contact lenses to:

- Registered opticians.
- Registered medical practitioners.
- Recognised medical students.

In addition, the General Optical Council was required to make regulations covering the fitting of contact lenses by training opticians and to submit these for approval to the Privy Council. The final sub-section of the new rules dealt with the penalties for contravening these regulations.

In June 1985 SI 1985/886 was published as 'The General Optical Council (Rules on the Fitting of Contact Lenses) Order of Council 1985'. The rules specified those groups of opticians in addition to those already qualified who may fit contact lenses as:

- Opticians engaged in approved basic training.
- Pre-registration students.
- Holders of partially recognized overseas qualifications who have concluded supplementary training in the United Kingdom.
- Those engaged in training for a higher contact lens qualification.

The rules also required that for any groups outlined above, contact lenses could only be fitted if under the continuous personal supervision of a registered optician or registered medical practitioner.

What Qualifications are required?

The Contact Lens (Qualifications, etc.) Rules 1988 (SI 1988/1305) issued by the General Optical Council to cover registrants fitting contact lenses came into force on 1 September 1988. Under the terms of the regulations, a registered optician was not allowed to fit a contact lens without either:

- An approved qualification.
- Certification.
- Provisional certification, or
- Adequate supervision.

A list of approved qualifications was published in Appendix A of the new rules as amended by SI 1989/375. The regulations meant that any newly qualified optometrist was entitled to fit lenses by virtue of having passed the contact lens examination section of the pre-qualifying examinations. Dispensing opticians, on the other hand, were required to take a supplementary examination to achieve an approved qualification. The regulations also removed the right of optometrists who qualified before 1960 to fit contact lenses without obtaining certification. The date of 1960 is chosen as the first date at which contact lenses were examined for qualification as a registered optometrist. The date appeared earlier in Notice N10 of the GOC in relation to annotation in the register.

To obtain certification an applicant had to show:

- Evidence of holding an approved qualification
- Evidence of having fitted a minimum of 150 patients in the previous 3 years
- Current involvement in teaching contact lens practice and evidence of involvement for at least 3 years in the full-time instruction of persons training as opticians in an approved training institution.

It was possible also to obtain professional certification if a registered optometrist:

- Anticipated that they would have fitted contact lenses to at least 150 persons in the period September 1986 to September 1989
- Was undertaking, or about to undertake, a course of study leading, after examination, to an approved qualification.

The final cut-off date for those not meeting the new requirements was 31 December 1990. This move prompted considerable anger from practitioners who qualified before 1960, the argument against the new Rules being that they removed an existing right that such practitioners had to fit lenses. The General Optical Council tried to make certification as straightforward as possible for those affected and the British College of Optometrists obtained General Optical Council approval to set a supplementary examination in contact lenses for optometrists falling outside the scope of SI 1988/1305.

What is a contact lens specification?

The Contact Lens Specification Rules 1989 (SI 1989/791) were introduced to provide an opportunity for patients to obtain contact lenses from any appropriate source and not just the practice at which the fitting took place. According to these rules the optometrist fitting the lenses must give the patient a written contact lens specification immediately following the final fitting (although what constitutes final fitting has not been defined). The information provided in the specification must be adequate to allow replication of the lens by another person and according to The Opticians Act 1989 (Amendment) Order 2005 SI 2005 No. 848 must include the following particulars:

- the name and address of the individual;
- if the individual has not attained the age of sixteen on the day the specification is issued the date of birth;
- the name and registration number of the person signing the specification;
- the address from which the person signing the specification practices;
- the name of the practice on whose premises the fitting took place;
- the date the fitting was completed;
- sufficient details of any lens fitted to enable a person who fits or supplies a contact lens to replicate the lens;
- the date the specification expires; and such information of a clinical nature as the person fitting the lens considers to be necessary in the particular case.

The exception initially was that an optometrist would not be required to supply information to an optician who was not qualified to fit contact lenses under the provision of SI1988/1305. This however was later updated to allow anyone to supply contact lenses against a valid specification.

The advent of internet services meant that patients were able to purchase lenses from non-clinical sources if they were provided to the specification that a clinician had issued. Often these lenses were considered by the patient as being cheaper but included no provision for after-care. The GOC still believed it was the duty of a practitioner to ensure the continuing clinical well-being of the patient, but this was obviously extremely difficult if the patient could purchase lenses and solutions elsewhere. The practitioner had a duty to inform a patient when after care was due but if the patient was purchasing lenses elsewhere and failed to attend how would that work? It was considered normal to attempt to recall a patient more than once for aftercare but if there was no response the practitioner was advised to contact the patient in writing indicating that without aftercare no responsibility could be taken for any damage that occurred to the eyes due to contact lens wear and that the contact lens specification would become out of date.

Trial lens fitting

The autumn of 1999 saw changes to the way contact lens practitioners fitted lenses. For some time, it had been shown that there was a small risk of variant Creutzfeldt- Jacob Disease being transmitted via corneal transplant. In late 1999 the Government Advisory committee on the disease (SEAC) decided that there was also a risk of transmission via contact lenses. There had been no reported cases and no contaminated contact lenses had been found but in response to the report the Medical Devices Agency introduced advice preventing the re-use of trial contact lenses. It also warned against the use of contact devices for measuring intra-ocular pressure without adequate precautions (disposable equipment being recommended). Following the MDA decision, the General Optical Council advised that the re-use of trial contact lenses introduced a risk of infection and should therefore be abandoned.

The latest position on contact lenses is covered by The Opticians Act 1989, The Opticians Act 1989 (Amendment) Order 2005 (S.I. 2005/848), and The General Optical Council (Injury or Disease of the Eye and

Contact Lens (Qualifications)) (Amendment) Rules Order of Council 2005 SI 2005 No. 1476.

The regulations as laid out in the Opticians Act specify that contact lenses (CLs) can only be fitted by an optometrist, contact lens optician (CLO) or registered medical practitioner. There are exceptions for people undertaking training. Section 25(9) of the Act defines "Fitting" as *"assessing whether a contact lens meets the needs of the individual; and, where appropriate providing the individual with one or more contact lenses for use during a trial period"*.

The fitting process

Before being fitted with contact lenses a patient should have been provided with enough information to be able to make an informed choice as to whether to go ahead. The information provided should include the risks and complications of wearing contact lenses and the potential consequences of not complying with advice on how to wear and care for contact lenses safely, the advantages and disadvantages of available contact lens types including advice on those that would be most appropriate and available care systems and risks of non-compliance with general contact lens related hygiene and replacement schedules. College of Optometrist guidance (Section A348) advises that to conduct an adequate assessment an optometrist should:

- include any additional tests indicated by:
  o symptoms
  o ocular and medical history
  o pre-disposing factors
- ask for, and consider, relevant information about:
  o history of allergies, including to components of contact lenses or their care products
  o history of systemic disease
  o previous contact lens wear
  o occupational and recreational needs
  o the environments in which contact lenses will be worn

- carry out a detailed assessment of the anterior eye which might be affected by wearing contact lenses. This should include:
  o a slit-lamp examination
  o keratometry or corneal topography
  o the use of diagnostic stains
  o the assessment of tear film quality and quantity
  o other factors, including the patient's ability to handle and care for the contact lenses safely and hygienically
- discuss with the patient why they are considered unsuitable for contact lens wear, if this is the case
- record all relevant information in the patient notes.

Once fitting is completed as mentioned above the patient must be given a copy of their contact lens specification and be provided with an appropriate lens care regimen, given adequate instruction on the use and wear of lenses, and provided with instructions and information on the care, wearing, treatment, cleaning and maintenance of the lens or lenses. (See the Opticians Act 1989 s 25[5][b]).

A patient should not be 'fitted' with contact lenses unless they have had a recent sight test, and this requirement would include when returning for check-ups at which a specification is re-affirmed or changed as that action is considered as effectively 'fitting' them (again) with contact lenses.

Supply of contact Lenses

Supply of contact lenses is also covered by regulation and there is a subtle distinction made between supply of powered contact lenses and supply of plano contact lenses. Powered contact lenses, according to S.27 of the Act, can only be supplied against a valid prescription by or under the supervision or general direction of an optometrist, dispensing optician, or medical practitioner (s.27(1)(b) and 27(3)(d)) and if they are for a person who is under 16, they cannot be sold under general direction (i.e., it must be direct supply or supply under supervision).

Plano contact lenses however can only be supplied by or under the supervision of an optometrist, dispensing optician, or medical practitioner (s.27(1)(b)) and the supervisor must be on the premises and able to exercise their professional skill and judgement as a clinician therefore they cannot be supplied under general direction.

In this instance the College of Optometrists Guidance (Section A393) offers the following on what is expected when supervising someone who is supplying the contact lens:

- *there should be written procedures in place to protect patients' health and safety*
- *the person supplying should have full understanding of the respective roles and responsibilities*
- *the person supplying is trained in the procedures to be followed*
- *the supervisor is on the premises and can intervene in the supply, if necessary*
- *the supervisor is in a position to exercise professional skill and judgement as a clinician*
- *arrangements are made for the patient to receive aftercare*
- *a sufficient audit trail is present so that any errors that occur can be drawn to the attention of the supervising optometrist*

The term general direction in relation to contact lens supply enables less rigorous systems to be established for supply that do not require direct supervision. For the system to operate the supplier must have one of the following:

- the original specification
- a copy of the specification
- a written or electronic order from the patient, which contains the details that are in the specification.
- If the original specification is not provided, then the details must be verified with whoever issued the specification.

Whilst the registrant responsible for general direction does not need to be on the premises during a sale, according to College of Optometrist guidelines to meet regulations they should ensure that:

- *written protocols and robust procedures are in place for verification and supply and to protect patient health and safety as far as is reasonable*
- *that the patient is not sight impaired, severely sight impaired or under 16*
- *the patient is not supplied with contact lenses which will take them past the expiry date of their specification*
- *they are a manager, or are in a position of authority to monitor the effectiveness of these protocols, and can make amendments to them if required*
- *there is an audit trail that can be followed*
- *the person conducting the supply is appropriately trained and they:*
  - *have working knowledge of the types of contact lenses available, the different care regimes and the replacement schedules for various lens types*
  - *can ensure that the contact lenses meet the specification*
  - *can advise the patient what to do if they suffer an adverse incident from the use of contact lenses or care solutions*
  - *tell the patient about the arrangements that are made for them to receive aftercare*
- *the person conducting the supply does not interpret or make judgements in relation to any clinical information in the specification and that they refer such matters to, and seek direction from, a registered optometrist, dispensing optician or doctor*

This was summarised in a paper by Hirji and Clarkson in 2007 which states *"General direction in this context was described during the passage of the legislation through Parliament as meaning that a registered practitioner is employed in the management chain of the supplier's business and accountable for what goes on between the supplier and the purchaser, ultimately answerable to the GOC therefore providing a measure of protection to the public hitherto absent. The seller (whether registered or unregistered) must also make reasonable arrangements for the person who is purchasing the contact lenses from the seller to receive aftercare."*

Plano Contact lens supply

Due to an increase in the sale of plano cosmetic contact lenses through unregulated outlets (particularly cosmetic designs to change the appearance of the eye) in 2017 the GOC produced a guide "**Do you know the law on selling contact lenses**?" The guidance was aimed at the unregistered suppliers particularly those supplying cosmetic lenses and spelled out the current legal framework as shown below:

"The sale of cosmetic contact lenses is covered by law

The Opticians Act covers the sale of zero-powered cosmetic and novelty contact lenses, used to change the colour or appearance of the eyes, as well as contact lenses that people wear to correct their vision. This is because using contact lenses that are unsuitable for the eyes, or using them incorrectly, can cause serious damage including, in extreme cases, blindness.

Are you breaking the law?

- *Zero-powered cosmetic contact lenses can be supplied only under the supervision of a registered optometrist, dispensing optician or medical practitioner.*
- *"Supervision" means that the registered person is present on the premises, in a position to oversee the work undertaken and ready to intervene if necessary.*
- *The seller/supplier must also make arrangements for the wearer to receive ongoing care.*
- *Any sales of cosmetic contact lenses that do not meet these requirements are illegal under the Opticians Act."*

Tackling illegal practice is not a statutory function of the GOC and although it may be considered as part of the wider remit to protect the public there is no mechanism for this. The internet represents a particular challenge because although the UK's laws on contact lens supply are among the strictest in the world many websites not complying with UK law and supplying lenses to UK patients are based in other countries with looser regulation. The Foresight report (see Chapter 8) discusses potential legal issues relating to overseas supply of products in the future as technology develops.

As supply of cosmetic lenses by unregistered sellers is a criminal offence in breach of the regulations where illegal sellers are UK-based the GOC can consider prosecution in line with the GOC protocol for investigating and prosecuting criminal offences. To do this however the GOC must weigh up the potential risk to patients and would only proceed where it was considered warranted.

Chapter 12

Referral, Record Keeping and Data Protection

Patient referral is one of the most important functions of the optometrist in routine practice. Optometrists act as effective eye care providers by opportunistically detecting and sending for further investigation those patients with ocular abnormalities and monitoring/managing those patients identified with a condition that is not yet ready for treatment. This screening and monitoring process has proved to be efficient, effective, and successful and has slowly been incorporated into the local health management processes for eyecare.

Referral by optometrists is for the most part covered by 2 sets of regulation:

1. The GOC rules relating to injury or disease of the eye
2. The GOS contract requirements

GOC Rules on referral

The GOC in fulfilment of the duty laid on them under s.31(5) of the Opticians Act first made rules relating to injury or disease of the eye in 1960 and produced guidance notes at that time in their N22 publication. These rules were in effect until the current Regulations SI1999/3267 were introduced. The GOC has defined the terms, "injury or disease", as used initially in the Opticians Act 1958 and repeated in the Opticians Act 1989, to cover conditions that cause or are likely to cause detriment to health or sight but excluding variations of refraction or normal changes due to age.

According to the current rules (as outlined in Chapter 7) where it appears to a registered optician that a person consulting him is suffering from an injury or disease of the eye normally the patient should be referred to a registered medical practitioner. In addition, where a patient has been directed by a medical practitioner to have an assessment (other than a recommendation for a sight test) a report should be sent back to that practitioner containing findings of any injury or disease of the eye of which the practitioner may be unaware.

The GOC rules state that when making a referral a registered optometrist should advise the person to consult a medical practitioner (this may be a GP or consultant) and wherever practicable provide a written report of findings indicating the grounds for thinking the person may be suffering from injury or disease of the eye. Where action appears urgent an optometrist should take appropriate action and where possible inform the patient's medical practitioner immediately. The developments in triage systems and co-management pathways have somewhat overtaken the regulations and the GOC in the issued Standards for Practice for Optometrists state more broadly in section 7.2 *Provide or arrange any further examinations, advice, investigations or treatment if required for your patient*. This should be done in a timescale that does not compromise patient safety and care.

If having advised a patient who appears to be suffering from injury or disease of the eye to consult a practitioner the patient is unwilling, on conscientious or other grounds to take the advice then that fact and the grounds which the person gives for unwillingness to consult a registered medical practitioner should be included on the patient record. This is essential for practitioners to safeguard against future potential claims and to fulfil audit requirements.

If an optometrist in their professional judgement considers there is no justification for the patient to be referred or it would be impracticable or inexpedient to make a referral they may decide not to refer and, in that event, should record:

- a sufficient description of the injury or disease from which that person appears to be suffering
- the reason for deciding not to refer on that occasion
- details of any advice offered to the patient and
- if appropriate, and with the consent of the patient, inform that person's general medical practitioner of those matters recorded.

The GOC Rules do not prevent a registered optician from providing, in an emergency, whatever services are in the best interests of the patient including treatment in accordance with rules in section 31 of the Opticians Act however notes of any actions should always be recorded. This situation is increasingly common in practice with the development of independent prescribing qualifications and NHS commissioned services.

Failure to comply with these rules could lead to a case being brought before the Fitness to Practice Committee of the GOC, and if proven could lead to erasure of the optometrist's name from the Register.

GOS contract requirements on referral

The NHS Terms of Service initially contained details on referral, and these were embodied in SI 1986/975 and amended by SI 1989/1175. However, although little changed in the detail the introduction of the new GOS contract in 2008 saw a duty placed on a contractor to ensure that action was taken by performers offering GOS with regard to patient referral.

The contract specifies that once a contractor has accepted a patient for GOS sight testing the duties identified in section 26 of the Opticians Act apply. Where a contractor or an optometrist employed by the contractor performs the GOS sight test and is of the opinion that a patient whose sight was tested shows on examination signs of injury, disease, or abnormality in the eye or elsewhere which may require medical treatment or is not able to attain a satisfactory standard of vision even with corrective lenses the patient should be referred. Referral may be to a general practitioner or to an ophthalmic hospital, which includes an ophthalmic department of a hospital and inform the patient's doctor or GP practice. Referral however should only take place with the consent of the patient and the patient should be provided with written details of the referral.

As optometric practice and training has developed several schemes have been established within the NHS that contract with optometrists either to provide a management service to prevent unnecessary/inappropriate referrals or to route patients via a triage system. As IT systems develop there is greater integration within eye care services and IT links allow video triage of patients by consultant led virtual clinics saving time resources by reducing inappropriate referrals and patient worry by providing rapid feedback on potential referrals.

These contractual regulations relate to a contractor or optometrist providing or performing GOS sight testing under contract to NHS England or participating in additional contractual arrangements with local commissioners. Failure to comply with these rules could lead to disciplinary action by NHS England and, ultimately, withdrawal of the contractor's or performer's name from the appropriate list.

It is generally considered that, under SI 1999/3267, the optometrist transfers the authority for dealing with a patient to the general practitioner upon referral. At one time this was interpreted as meaning that the general practitioner should decide whether spectacles should be prescribed and be able to intercept if required. In modern practice this is an unrealistic situation as patients may wait for a significant period for a non-urgent GP appointment and longer for a hospital appointment but can be supplied with spectacles within one hour.

In an emergency, for example, where a patient is unable to follow his occupation or is gravely inconvenienced without spectacles the optometrist has always been able to make the decision to supply spectacles provided that this is unlikely to prevent the patient from seeking further advice. There is no evidence that GPs are advising that spectacles have been provided inappropriately where the provision of spectacles would be appropriate and in the best interests of the patient. If spectacles are supplied when a patient is referred, then it should be made clear to the patient that the spectacles are supplied on a provisional basis and that the prescription may need to be modified following the outcome of any referral and a suitable note should be included on the patient record.

General referral procedures

With the advent of modern technology and the introduction of secure NHS email links for optometrists often a patient referral will be made by email direct to a GP practice or consultant. The use of fax has been phased out due to issues with General Data Protection requirements and levels of security. However, it is still considered acceptable for the optometrist to post a letter to the GP or give the patient a letter to deliver by hand to their general medical practitioner.

There is a requirement under the GOS contract to supply the patient with a written copy of the referral details for their own records (the exception would be where it could be considered harmful to the patient if they were aware of the full content).

Information-only referrals

Following the abolition of Form OSC1 (used by general practitioners to refer patients to an optometrist when the NHS was established), the optometrist had been expected, out of courtesy, to write to the general practitioner in certain situations that would not constitute a referral. This form of contact with a patient's GP is now used to notify them either of a condition of which they may not be aware or where an optometrist has identified a condition but decided to monitor/manage rather than refer. The notification enables the GP to update the patient record.

Layout of referral letters

Referral should be made either by submission of an appropriate GOS 18 form, or on headed notepaper showing the practice address. When using headed notepaper, the letter should be dated and should begin with the patient's full name and address. It should contain details of history and symptoms, vision, and visual correction with best acuities for distance and near, together with any previous acuities and the date recorded. The reasons for referral (e.g., motility problems, poor acuity, fundus abnormality) should be clearly stated. Finally, the letter must be signed by the referring optometrist and a duplicate retained with the patient's record and a copy should be provided to the patient or if the patient does not want a copy note this on the record card. The GOS18 form is a standard NHS form that is reviewed periodically to take account of changes in practice. When using a GOS18 all appropriate sections should be completed. There is a requirement to indicate the level of urgency of a referral to assist with ensuring a patient receives the most timely and appropriate care. In cases where a triaging/electronic referral system operates there may be specific referral documentation that forms part of the process, and it is important that the correct form is completed to prevent delays.

Clinical Case records

This is an area of practice that receives far less attention than it deserves. The NHS requires contractors (and therefore performers) to maintain clear accurate and contemporaneous records. It is the case record that provides for continuing care of a patient and can make or break the outcome of a Fitness to Practise or NHS investigation and hearing. Despite all the changes in technology and the extensive introduction of computerised records it is sad to say that some practice records both electronic and hard copy still fall below an adequate standard. It is likely that most practitioners would not consider that they themselves are inadequate record keepers but this section, by outlining the bare minimum contents and demonstrating the essential elements of a record, may make them think again.

The Quality in Optometry website offers a helpful audit tool for assessing the content of clinical records and there is a minimum expected standard for GOS clinical sight test records both of which are useful in assessing standard of record keeping. The GOC have indicated that failure to keep acceptable and adequate records may be considered to constitute serious professional misconduct. Indeed, there have been cases in which the GOC have made an erasure order on the basis of poor record keeping. Included in the GOC standards of practice, standard 8 requires an optometrist to "Maintain adequate patient records" and includes the following as the minimum expected:

- The date of the consultation.
- A patient's personal details.

- The reason for the consultation and any presenting condition.
- The details and findings of any assessment or examination conducted.
- Details of any treatment, referral or advice provided, including any drugs or optical device prescribed or a copy of a referral letter.
- Consent obtained for any examination or treatment.
- Details of all those involved in the optical consultation, including name and signature, or other identification of the author.

The College of Optometrists guidelines offer additional advice on the content of a patient record expected for a reasonable optometrist.

Records are intended to carry information pertinent to the patient's problems. They also act as a note to a practitioner of findings from an earlier examination and provide a means of evaluating change in basic measurements. It is always sensible to quickly review at least the previous record when seeing a patient. The exact style of the record card is left to the individual practitioner although in the case of computerisation companies produce their own template. Records vary from simply blank cards (although these are becoming far less common) to electronic systems providing enough space to include detailed personal (non-clinical) information such as what the patient is hoping to do for a holiday so that this can be recollected at the next visit to provide a personal touch — this has to be done with care however so as not to breach General Data Protection requirements!

A potential risk with electronic records is the "Pre-populating" of fields that occurs in some systems. This fills in information before the patient has been seen taking it from the previous record and requiring the clinician to cancel the information that is no longer correct and replace with new. If the information is not updated, then the record data become invalid.

The use of two systems in tandem (a paper system and a computerised system) can also cause issues with information shared between different sources and not comprehensive on both. It is recognised that changing from paper base to computer will require a managed period of scanning old records etc but where a new computerized system is introduced ALL records after the date of introduction should be on the new system and all performers should be using the new system. In situations where each practitioner may use a different system i.e., one using paper and one using electronic the risk of error is increased significantly.

Whatever the style of the record to be used in line with professional guidance the following basic details are expected to be included.

Personal details of the patient

Name: There are few records that do not carry the patient's name. It is important, however, that the full name is recorded and not just initials. From a filing point of view, it can be an absolute nightmare trying to locate a Mrs Smith without the first and second names. It is worth noting that patients do not always call themselves by their first name and it is useful to have a system that allows for this either by insisting on the correct first name being on the record or by having a cross referencing system particularly as a patient frequently forgets the information they have given at a previous test.

Address: This also is essential and should be updated whenever the patient points out a change.

Telephone number: It helps immensely if a patient can be reached by telephone during the day. For example, if something goes wrong with the promised job, you can advise the patient before the patient has to chase you. It is also becoming more common for patients to be comfortable with receiving appointment reminders by text.

Date of birth: The full date of birth is particularly important where, for example, father and son have the same names and live at the same address.

Date of examination: There is nothing more irritating for a clinician who asks for the date of the last examination than to be told "Oh, it was little while ago". From a legal standpoint, the date of examination could be an important factor in deciding whether a condition should have been noted at that time and should always be accurately recorded. It is also an important factor in NHS audit to determine intervals between sight tests.

Occupation: It is usually necessary to know the patient's occupation to assist with prescribing. If glasses are prescribed for a specific occupation, they may prove totally unsuitable if the patient decides to change jobs.

General practitioner's name and address: This information should be recorded for two reasons. First, it is needed for referral letters; secondly, if, as sometimes happens, a health clinic contacts the practice to ask for information about a patient, you are able to check with whom you are dealing.

Hobbies: This information is necessary to help with the best choice of correction when prescribing.

Clinical details of the patient

Ocular history: Has the patient had an eye examination previously? If so, were spectacles prescribed and, if so, for what were they to be used? Has the patient ever had any eye injury or operation and, if so, what was its nature and when? Are any ocular medications being used?

Symptoms: Why has the patient decided to visit an optometrist? Do they suffer from eye ache or headaches? When do the symptoms occur etc? Does the patient have flashes or floaters?

General health: Is the patient suffering from any general disorder or taking tablets, pills, or other medication? If yes full details should be recorded?

Family history: Is there any history of eye problems or of general health problems that may affect the eyes in the family?

Examination details

Unaided vision or (if available) the visual acuities with existing spectacles (distance and near) is better to enable assessment of the benefits of any observed/proposed prescription change

Autorefractor/retinoscopy as an objective refractive assessment
Subjective refractive result to be prescribed
Best corrected distance visual acuity
Oculomotor Balance information
Near reading correction (if necessary) and acuity achieved at near (with working distance if outside "normal" expectation)
External examination of the eyes

Internal examination of the eyes. It is important that the patient record shows that a full examination has been carried out. An adequate record would be expected to include information such as:

- media clear
- discs flat
- disc margins clear
- disc pallor
- cup/disc ratio 0.3
- fundus clear and healthy
- Artery/Vein ratio 2/3
- Macula clear

this shows that the individual structures were examined, and clinical observations made on each. The use of ticks, abbreviations and arrows should be avoided. With the advent of imaging and Optical Coherence Tomography it is particularly important to ensure that the observations recorded are consistent with the images stored.

Supplementary tests

Details of any supplementary tests carried out and the outcome should be recorded — this is particularly important if there is a change from previous test results. It is also important where for example a field plot is printed that this is signed off by the clinician and kept with the patient record or linked to the patient record.

Action taken

A decision on "patient disposal" should include for example type of lenses advised and when they should be used, a copy of any referral note with comment if the patient is advised to visit the general practitioner, suggested recall interval and reason if less than a standard period and the patient's signature if advice is rejected.

Examiner's name

The examiner's name should be identifiable from the record to ensure that should any problems or queries arise the most appropriate individual can respond.

The above outline simply presents basic type of information required and should not be considered as exhaustive; it does not offer a layout and it does not offer any advice on the relative importance of each category. The College of Optometrists provides guidance on record content that can be found on the College website and was updated in 2021 and NHS England have produced advice on what would be expected from an NHS perspective as a minimum on case records.

Complete and accurate case records are a simple and effective way of providing best patient care and protecting clinical reputation. It is important that records are retained in line with data protection and there are minimum requirements for retention for NHS GOS patients. All GOS records should be retained for a minimum of seven years and there is a recommendation from professional bodies to maintain records for adults and deceased patients for 10 years from their last visit and for children until their 25th birthday. It important to stress again that retention of records is carried out in compliance with data protection requirements.

Data Protection and health records

Data protection is a complex subject, and the following is provided as guidance, but it is sensible to seek legal advice or advice from a professional body if there are any concerns about sharing data.

Requirements for data protection were controlled in the UK in 1984 via the Data Protection Act and this introduced the concept of an Information Commissioner (originally Registrar) responsible for the service. Anyone using personal data was (and still is) required to register with the Information Controller's Office (ICO) and to meet specific standards.

This Act was updated by the Data Protection Act 1998 and this Act in turn was repealed in 2018 and replaced by a new Data Protection Act 2018. The new Act was introduced in response to the European Union (General Data Protection requirements (Council Decision (EU) 2018/893)). The EU had published the relevant regulations as *Regulation (EU) 2016/679 of the European Parliament and of the Council of 27 April 2016 on the protection of natural persons with regard to the processing of personal data and on the free movement of such data (General Data Protection Regulation)*

For optical services in addition to the data protection requirements the Access to Health Records Act 1990 was laid before Parliament in July 1990 and came into force on 1 November 1991 impacting on patient access to health care information retained by a clinician. It was drafted to establish a right of access to health records by the individuals to whom the records relate and to certain others and to provide for the correction of inaccurate health records and remains in place with some amendments. Essentially it enables patients to ensure that any information held about them is correct and accurate and provides a system for modification of a record if it is shown to be incorrect.

The Data Protection requirements caused amendment to the Access to Health Records Act, and both sit comfortably side by side but there are differences. Under the terms of the 1990 Act a health record is defined as a record which:

- consists of information relating to the physical or mental health of an individual who can be identified from that information or from that and other information in the possession of the holder of the record, and
- has been made by or on behalf of a health professional in connection with the care of the individual.

The data protection Act is much broader in its definition of what is covered and describes personal data (including data relating to health) as:

"Any information relating to an identified or identifiable natural person ("data subject"); an identifiable person is someone who can be identified, directly or indirectly, in particular by reference to an identifier such as a name, an identification number, location data, online identifier or to one or more factors specific to the physical, physiological, genetic, mental, economic, cultural or social identity of that person."

Data Holder

Under the 1990 Act the holder of a record is defined as any 'health professional' that is included in this meaning within the Data Protection Act 1998 (amended to read the DPA 2018 on repeal of the 1998 Act).

The Data Protection Act has a different approach to holding data and defines a Data controller as:

"the person(s) or organisation that determines the purpose and means of processing personal data. In optics this would usually be the practice owner or company registered with the Information Commissioner but maybe someone appointed by the practice or business owner who has overall control and responsibility for how personal data is collected, processed and stored in a practice/business"

and a Data processor as:

"the person(s) or organisation(s) responsible for processing personal data on behalf of the controller (other than a person who is an employee of the controller)". This would relate to external service providers who have access to personal data to fulfil their role. Data processors are all other persons who process personal data on behalf of the controller (other than a person who is an employee of the controller). In an optical practice this could include a practice management software provider or payroll company, for example. It is also likely to include locums.

The data controller is responsible for ensuring that personal data is:

- processed lawfully, fairly, and transparently
- collected and used for specific and legitimate purposes, and not used in an incompatible way with those purposes
- adequate, relevant, and limited to what is necessary for the intended purposes
- accurate and where necessary kept up to date — e.g., errors can be rectified without undue delay
- kept in a way that permits identification of an individual for no longer than is necessary
- kept secure using appropriate technical or organizational measures — e.g., protecting against accidental loss, destruction, or damage.

Impact of Data Protection Act 2018 on optometry

As data protection has been built into the optical services for some time the new regulations had little major impact and were designed to strengthen citizens' rights by putting more focus on demonstrating data security and clearer accountability. One change however that has impacted on optical working practices was that all GOS providers became classified as public authorities and were therefore required to appoint a Data Protection Officer (DPO). The role of the DPO is to ensure that the organisation processes the personal data of its staff, patients/(customers), providers or any other individuals (also referred to as data subjects) in compliance with the applicable data protection rules. Article 39 of the original EU General Data Protection Regulations (GDPR) framework outlines the responsibilities and tasks of a DPO and the key areas these refer to may be summarised as:

- Educate the organisation and employees on important compliance requirements
- Train staff on what is required to process data securely
- Conduct spot-checks and audits to ensure compliance with GDPR
- Address non-compliance, or potential security breaches proactively
- Act as the primary point of contact between the organisation and the GDPR supervisory authorities

- Keep detailed records of all data processing activities conducted by the business, which includes a detailed explanation of the purpose of all processing activities, which the DPO must make public on request
- Inform 'data subjects' about how their data is being used, their rights to have their personal data erased and explain what measures the organisation has put in place to protect their personal information

This is quite daunting for a small optical business, but the Information Commissioner's Office (ICO) has been clear that the knowledge and expertise that the DPO is required to have should be proportionate to the type of processing carried out and the level of risk. It has recognised that small organisations may find it difficult to identify (or may not have) an employee who has both the skills to take on the role, and no potential conflict of interest with their other duties as an employee and therefore has indicated that it will be pragmatic when dealing with such cases, and that if an optical practice appoints a DPO with a potential conflict of interest then the practice should document the reasons for the appointment, what the possible conflicts of interest, are and what measures (if any) will be taken to reduce or eliminate such conflicts.

Information Commissioner

Most organisations that process personal information (and optical practices are no different) are required by law to register with the Information Commissioner. It is essential that all eye care providers therefore register and keep adequate patient records, comply with the Data Protection legislation, and understand responsibilities under the Freedom of Information Act. All individual optometrists even when not the "Record holder" as defined above have responsibilities to comply with the Data Protection Act and, from 25 May 2018, the EU General Data Protection Regulations (GDPR) and updated Data Protection Act 2018 (DPA 2018).

It is therefore important to be familiar with the Act and GDPR and the key elements for optometrists are:

- keeping accurate patient data
- using the data for specific purposes
- amending inaccurate data and responding to objections from patients if the use of the data causes harm or distress
- keeping the data no longer than necessary.
- keeping the data confidential and secure.
- enabling patients, or an applicant acting on behalf of a patient, to access their data for the length of time that the records are kept. It is important to verify that the applicant has a right to see the data, either because they have written authority from the patient or because they have Power of Attorney. Access to the record must be given within the time limit set out in the Act and the GDPR requires that if a patient asks for a copy of their record, this must be provided free of charge in most instances
- assisting the patient to understand their record by explaining its content and abbreviations
- satisfying yourself that there is no further need of the record before destroying it
- disposing of any records securely, and
- being aware that, if a patient record is acquired, the obligations under the Data Protection Act and GDPR transfer to you as the new owner.

Right of access

Under s. 3 of the Access to Health Records Act 1990 a request for access to the record or to any part of the record could be made to the record holder by:

- The patient.
- A person authorized in writing to make the application on the patient's behalf e.g., solicitor.
- Where the record is held in England and Wales and the patient is a child, a person having parental responsibility for the patient.
- Where the record is held in Scotland and the patient is a pupil, a parent or guardian of the patient.

- Where the patient is incapable of managing his own affairs, any person appointed by a court to manage those affairs.
- Where the patient has died, the patient's personal representative and any person who may have a claim arising out of the patient's death.

However subsequent regulations on data protection in 1998 and 2018 amended the Act by repealing items 1 to 5 leaving only clause 6 active. Currently access is given to a patient, or a third party who has been authorised by the patient, anyone who has a legal basis for access or where the patient has died, the patient's personal representative and any person who may have a claim arising out of the patient's death. Any request for access is classed as a subject access request (SAR). Rights of access are not confined to health records held by NHS bodies and apply equally to the private health sector and to health professionals' private practice records. Subject to the conditions explained in this guidance, individuals have a right to apply for access to health records irrespective of when they were compiled. Under Data Protection legislation Health and care records are confidential so can only be accessed by someone authorised to do so.

A person with parental responsibility will usually be entitled to access the records of a child who is aged 12 or younger. However, children aged 13 or older are usually considered to have the capacity to give or refuse consent to parents requesting access to their health records, unless there is a reason to suggest otherwise. In this latter situation however, every reasonable effort should be made to encourage the child to involve parents or guardians.

Copies of records which are supplied under subject access rights must be accompanied by an explanation of any terms that might be unintelligible to the patient or the person requesting access to the records. Even in cases where permanent copies cannot be supplied, an explanation of such terms is required.

Correction of records

Data protection regulations include a right for individuals to have inaccurate personal data rectified or completed if it is incomplete.

Where a person considers that any information contained in a health record to which they have access is incorrect, misleading, or incomplete they may apply to the controller of the record verbally or in writing for correction to be made. On such an application the holder has one calendar month in which to respond to the request. As it is a requirement under the Acts to ensure accuracy in records maintained there should be no issue however in making accuracy corrections, but it is important to note that the term "information" when relating to a health record includes any expression of opinion about the patient.

Refusal of access

The circumstances in which refusal of access may be considered are where:

- it is likely to cause serious physical or mental harm to the patient or another person.
- it relates to a third party who has not given consent for disclosure (where that third party is not a health professional who has cared for the patient) and after considering the balance between the duty of confidentiality to the third party and the right of access of the applicant, the data controller concludes it is reasonable to withhold third party information.
- it is requested by a third party and, the patient had asked that the information be kept confidential, or the records are subject to legal professional privilege.
- it is restricted by order of the courts

Freedom of Information Act

As part of the GOS contract any provider of General Ophthalmic Services depending on location must comply with obligations under the:

- Freedom of Information Act 2000 (FOIA) — if you are based in England, Northern Ireland, or Wales

- Freedom of Information (Scotland) Act 2002 (FOISA) — if you are based in Scotland.

An NHS GOS provider is classified as a 'public authority' under FOIA and FOISA. In practical terms this means there must be in place a 'publication scheme' approved by the:

- UK's Information Commissioner's Office (ICO) if you are based in England, Northern Ireland, or Wales
- Scottish Information Commissioner if you are based in Scotland.

Practicalities

In practical terms the GOS contract requires that certain information related specifically to GOS must be proactively published and available upon request. The Freedom of Information Act 2000 was designed to promote openness and accountability amongst all organisations that receive public money. Since 1 January 2005 there has been a FOI obligation on NHS optical contractors to respond to requests about the NHS related information that they hold, and a right of access to that information subject to specific exemptions has been established in law.

What is covered?

In general terms the published information should cover:

- Details of the business, details of the registered personnel employed and where applicable the company registration number
- A list and details of the policies and procedures in place covering complaints, data protection and health and safety where appropriate
- Details of the services offered within the NHS umbrella and how they can be accessed including opening times for the practice(s)
- Other relevant information

Organisations within the optical sector — FODO, ABDO, AOP and the College of Optometrists — collectively have produced the following guidance documents to cover England, Wales, and Northern Ireland to help to understand the information that should be shared as part of the model publication scheme:

- *Sector specific guidance for GOS providers* including a template format
- *Freedom of Information Act (FOI): Model Publication Scheme* (2009)

Chapter 13

Fitness to Practise

Optometrists face two main potential reviews of their fitness to practise one involving their suitability to provide General Ophthalmic Services and the other their suitability to remain on the register (or in the case of a student registrant to study to enter the profession). Although the two processes may well interact, they have different outcomes. The NHS procedures relate to a contractor or performer having broken the terms of the NHS contract and/or regulatory requirements as laid down in the relevant statutory instruments and are dealt with in Chapter 5; the GOC procedures are much more far reaching and can relate to anything which may pertain to the fitness to practise of a registrant. The outcome of the two procedures is also different in that the NHS investigation may result in prohibiting an optometrist from offering or performing GOS or other NHS services while the GOC investigation may result in erasure of the practitioner's name from the register and total prohibition to practise. In both cases the outcome may be that conditions on the way an individual is able to practise are imposed.

Original Scope of the GOC disciplinary process

Following the introduction of the 1958 Opticians Act and in accordance with ss.14 to 23 of the Opticians Act 1989 and regulated by SI 1960/1934, SI 1960/1935, SI 1961/1239 and SI 1961/1933, the GOC were charged with investigating any breach of professional discipline as considered appropriate. Until 2005 two committees, established under the Opticians Act 1958, and maintained by the Opticians Act 1989 carried out the relevant functions: the Investigation Committee carried out the preliminary investigation, and the Disciplinary Committee considered sufficiently serious disciplinary cases referred to them by the Investigating Committee. In the case of a decision by the Disciplinary Committee to strike the name of a registered optician from the register, there existed the right of appeal against the decision, to the Judicial Committee of the Privy Council.

The jurisdiction of the GOC committees covered the following offences:

- A criminal offence, other than a trivial one, by a registered optician
- Infamous conduct in any professional respect by a registered optician
- Any offence by a body corporate under the terms of the Opticians Act
- Failure by a body corporate to observe the required conditions of enrolment
- Connivance by a body corporate at conduct leading to the erasure from the register of the name of a registered optician in its employ
- Breach of the rules made under s. 25 of the Opticians Act relating to:
  o Publicity
  o The name under which business is carried out
  o The administering of drugs
- The prescription, supply, and fitting of contact lenses
- Failure to make adequate arrangements for the fitting and supply of optical appliances
- Entries in a register made on fraudulent or incorrect grounds

Initial Composition of the Investigating Committee

When first established the Investigating Committee had no special procedure laid down and ordinary committee procedure applied. The Chairman of the GOC could not be a member of this committee. The Committee was made up of six members of Council, two of whom were lay members, one an ophthalmologist, two representatives of ophthalmic opticians and one a representative of dispensing opticians. If the dispensing representative declared an interest in a particular case, then the place was taken by either an ophthalmologist or a lay member of the Council. If the case was to be against a body corporate then the committee could co-opt either an ophthalmic representative or a dispensing representative of corporate bodies, depending upon the allegation.

Composition of the Disciplinary Committee

The procedure for the Disciplinary Committee was updated and set out in the General Optical Council (Disciplinary Committee) (Procedure) Order of Council 1985, SI 1985/1580 and revised by SI1998/1338. By 1998 the Committee consisted of 15 members of the Council appointed by the Council made up as follows:

1. Three members from among those appointed by the Privy Council one of which would be Chairman of the Committee
2. Two members from among the registered medical practitioners on Council
3. Four members from among those chosen to represent registered optometrists on Council
4. Three members from among those chosen to represent dispensing opticians on Council
5. Three further members from among those in the above categories not already selected

The quorum for a committee was five and included a member of the committee appointed under each of 2, 3 and 4 above. If members were unable to be present due to a specific conflict of interest a member of Council may be co-opted to the Committee to provide a quorum.

Should the Chairman of the Committee be absent when a disciplinary case was due for hearing the committee could elect one of its members present to preside as acting Chairman.

The committee was required to meet at least once a year and all meetings would normally have taken place at the GOC offices in London although this changed in 2001 when the offices of another professional body with better facilities was also used.

No person who had been on the Investigating Committee for a particular case could also sit on the Disciplinary Committee for that case.

Position by 2022

The format and procedure of disciplinary hearings changed significantly in 2005 when new Fitness to Practise (FTP) regulations were put in place via *The Opticians Act 1989 (Amendment) Order 2005 SI 2005/848*. These regulations were further amended by *The General Optical Council (Fitness to Practise) Rules Order of Council 2013 SI 2013/2537*. This latter change saw the introduction of case examiners whose role was to review complaints presented and determine whether any allegations made appeared serious enough to proceed to a full investigation. Each allegation was to be reviewed by 2 case examiners one of whom must be a lay person and the other either a registered dispensing optician or a registered optometrist depending on the case.

What are considered as potential FTP matters?

Currently according to the Opticians Act 1989 the following would be considered as areas where the fitness to practise of a registered optometrist or registered dispensing optician, or the fitness to undertake training of a student registrant, may be "impaired":

o   misconduct;
o   deficient professional performance (except in the case of a student registrant);
o   a conviction or caution in the British Islands for a criminal offence, or a conviction elsewhere for an offence which, if committed in England and Wales, would constitute a criminal offence;
o   the registrant having accepted a conditional offer under section 302 of the Criminal Procedure (Scotland) Act 1995 (fixed penalty: conditional offer by procurator fiscal) or agreed to pay a penalty under

section 115A of the Social Security Administration Act 1992 (penalty as alternative to prosecution);

o the registrant, in proceedings in Scotland for an offence, having been the subject of an order under section 246(2) or (3) of the Criminal Procedure (Scotland) Act 1995 discharging him absolutely;

o adverse physical or mental health; or

o a determination by a body in the United Kingdom responsible under any enactment for the regulation of a health or social care profession to the effect that an individual's fitness to practise as a member of that profession is impaired, or a determination by a regulatory body elsewhere to the same effect.

In the case of a business registrant the following areas would be considered where fitness to carry on business as an optometrist or a dispensing optician or to carry on both businesses may be impaired:

o misconduct by the business registrant or by one of its directors

o practices or patterns of behaviour occurring within the business which —
   –   the registrant knew or ought reasonably to have known of; and
   –   amount to misconduct or deficient professional performance

o the instigation by the business registrant of practices or patterns of behaviour within the business where that practice or behaviour amounts, or would if implemented amount, to misconduct or deficient professional performance

o a conviction or caution in the British Islands of the business registrant or one of its directors for a criminal offence, or a conviction elsewhere for an offence which, if committed in England or Wales, would constitute a criminal offence

o the registrant or one of its directors having accepted a conditional offer under section 302 of the Criminal Procedure (Scotland) Act 1995 or agreed to pay a penalty under section 115A of the Social Security Administration Act 1992

o the registrant or one of its directors, in proceedings in Scotland for an offence, having been the subject of an order under section 246(2) or (3) of the Criminal Procedure (Scotland) Act 1995 discharging it or him absolutely

o   a determination by a body in the United Kingdom responsible under any enactment for the regulation of a health or social care profession to the effect that
  (i) the business registrant's fitness to carry on business as a member of that profession is impaired; or
  (ii) the fitness of a director of the business registrant to practise that profession is impaired,
     or a determination by a regulatory body elsewhere to the same effect.

Within these areas references to a conviction include a conviction by court martial and an allegation may refer to acts or omissions that occurred outside the United Kingdom or at a time when the registrant was not registered.

The introduction of the new process in 2005 saw the GOC establish an independent panel of 38 members to participate in hearings the membership of which included lay, registrant and legal personnel. The panel members are collectively referred to as the Fitness to Practise Hearings Panel and form the Fitness to Practise Committee and the Registration Appeals Committee. They are not Council members. Both lay and professional members of the Hearings Panel are independent of the GOC and panel members are appointed for a term of five years, with the option to serve for a further five years on application. In every case against an optometrist or a dispensing optician, there will be a lay majority on the panel. A different hearings panel is selected for each hearing and each panel has a maximum of five people, chosen from the 38 members. All hearings are supported by a legal adviser. The current processes are laid out in the Fitness to Practice Rules 2013 *(The General Optical Council (Fitness to Practise) Rules Order of Council 2013 SI 2013/2537)*.

What is the process when an allegation is made?

Under the current system the Registrar of the GOC initially considers all matters concerning fitness to practice received by the GOC. The Registrar must consider patient safety and as a first stage whether to refer a matter directly to the FTP Committee for consideration as to whether an interim order should be made where risk is high. Also, it is the role of the Registrar to determine whether an allegation falls within one of the grounds described in section 13D of the Opticians Act, (listed above) if it does not then the Registrar notifies the complainant, and the case will be closed.

Where the Registrar considers that an allegation does fall within one or more of the grounds described in section 13D of the Opticians Act the allegation must be referred to case examiners for consideration — although further investigation and evidence gathering may have been undertaken by the GOC investigation team as part of the initial process. An exception to this is that where an allegation relates to a conviction that has resulted in a custodial sentence, whether immediate or suspended, the Registrar must refer the case to the FTP Committee.

Only a minority of the complaints that are made to the GOC result in a referral to the FTP Committee. In the majority of complaints, case examiners decide that there is no need for any further action to be taken or that the matter can be appropriately dealt with by issuing a registrant with a warning or advice. In 2018–19 for example only 17% of cases considered were referred to the FTP Committee.

Who are Case Examiners and how do they work?

The review in 2013 of the FTP processes resulted in the establishment of a panel of Case Examiners and the revised Fitness to Practise Rules (2013) define a case examiner as *"an officer of the Council appointed by the Registrar on the Council's behalf for the purposes of exercising the functions of the Investigation Committee (IC), in accordance with these rules, being a registered optometrist or dispensing optician, or a lay person."* The GOC has published guidance for case examiners.

All cases for investigation must be referred to two case examiners one a registered case examiner and one a lay case examiner. If at the end of the investigation stage, the case examiners do not agree on the outcome the matter will be referred to the Investigation Committee. When determining their outcome case examiners will be able to obtain independent legal advice and/or expert advice if it is felt necessary.

In determining an outcome following investigation of an allegation and in particular determining whether the case should be referred to the FTP Committee it is expected that the case examiners should ask themselves the following question:

"Is there a realistic prospect of establishing that the registrant's fitness to practise is impaired to a degree that justifies action being taken against their registration?"

This is known as "the realistic prospect test". All conclusions by the Case Examiners should be based on the "realistic prospect test" and they must remember that their role is not to make decisions on the facts (that is the function of the FTP Committee), but only to determine whether the realistic prospect test has been met.

When considering an allegation, case examiners may unanimously determine to close certain categories of case that, in the public interest, ought not to proceed through the fitness to practise procedure. The relevant categories of case are as follows:

- An allegation which arises from events which occurred more than five years before the matter was brought to the attention of the GOC, (except in exceptional circumstances)
- An allegation which is made by a complainant who wishes to remain anonymous or has indicated that they do not wish to co-operate further (although case examiners must bear in mind the GOC's own powers of investigation)
- Any allegation which the case examiners consider to be vexatious in nature.

Reasons for case examiner adjournments

Further investigation

If at any stage, prior to deciding the final outcome, case examiners request additional information then consideration of a case may be adjourned, and the Registrar informed. The Registrar will initiate the additional investigation and will provide any additional evidence obtained to the registrant and, where appropriate, to the maker of the allegation, giving them a reasonable opportunity to respond. The Registrar will then provide the case examiners with all additional evidence, together with any further comments to enable them to resume their consideration of the matter.

Additional potential allegations

Should case examiners consider that there may be evidence (either from the complaint made to the GOC or from any further investigation) of allegations not included initially by the Registrar, or that the allegations should be amended, the case examiners should adjourn consideration of the case and inform the Registrar. The matters raised and whether additional or alternative allegations should be drafted for consideration by the case examiners may be considered by the Registrar. After the registrant has had an opportunity to respond to any new or amended allegations/evidence the case examiners should resume their consideration of the matter.

Decision making by Case Examiners

When deciding an outcome about a particular allegation, case examiners will consider not only the original allegation, and any evidence that has been gathered by the GOC, but also any written representations that have been received from the registrant concerned and the maker of the allegation where appropriate. A registrant must be given copies of any information or documents received in support of the allegation and allowed 28 days in which to make any written representations before the case examiners consider the allegation(s).

What are the potential outcomes of the case examiners' considerations?

There are several potential outcomes arising from the case examiners' consideration of an allegation and these are:

- referral of the case to the FTP Committee
- referral to the Investigating Committee where the case examiners are unable to reach a unanimous decision
- the issue of a warning to the registrant
- a decision to take no further action including issuing a registrant with advice about their future conduct
- a decision to take no further action

The case examiners should always consider the public interest. The wider public interest includes not just the protection of members of the public, but the maintenance of public confidence in the profession, and the declaring and upholding of proper standards of conduct and behaviour. When referring a case to the FTP Committee consideration (in line with the realistic prospect test) is given to the following two issues:

- Is there a realistic prospect of being able to prove the facts alleged against the registrant, if the allegation is referred to the FTP Committee?
- If the alleged facts were proved, are they so significant as to indicate that the registrant's fitness to practice is or may be impaired to a degree that justifies action being taken against their registration

As mentioned earlier it is not the role of the case examiners to decide whether a registrant's fitness to practice is impaired — that is a decision for the FTP Committee to make (if the matter is referred). But in utilizing the realistic prospect test, the case examiners should have regard to the following:

- they should proceed with caution (given that case examiners are working from documents alone and the evidence before them may be untested);
- it is not the role of the case examiners to make any findings of fact. It is for the FTP Committee to make factual findings;
- the FTP Committee will only find facts disputed by the registrant proved if, having heard the evidence, the Committee considers it more likely than not to have happened (the "civil standard of proof");

However, the case examiners must not (normally) resolve substantial conflicts of evidence;

- where there is a plain conflict between two accounts, either one of which may realistically be correct, and on one account the matter would call into question the registrant's fitness to practice, the conflict should be resolved by the FTP Committee, not the case examiners;
- if case examiners are in doubt about whether to refer the matter to the FTP Committee, they should consider the complainant's version of events and then apply the realistic prospect test;
- it is not the case examiners' role to refer to the FTP Committee an allegation that is not supported by any evidence. There must be a genuine (not remote or fanciful) possibility both that the facts alleged could be found proved and that if they are, the registrant's fitness to practise could be found impaired by the FTP Committee
- when determining whether the realistic prospect test is met in relation to an allegation of culpable omission (i.e., that the registrant failed to do something that they should have done), the case examiners must consider whether
    o there is a realistic prospect of proving that the registrant had a duty to do the specified thing AND
    o that there is a realistic prospect of proving that the registrant failed to do the specified thing.
- If the realistic prospect test is not met for both it will not be met for the allegation overall
- there is a public interest in both business registrants and individual registrants not being harassed by unfounded allegations
- where the "realistic prospect" test is met, there is a public interest in there being a public hearing before the FTP Committee
- the case examiners should proceed with caution in reaching a decision not to refer a case where the decision may be perceived as inconsistent with a decision made by another public body (for example, a decision where there has been input from optical professionals, or a decision of an NHS body), in relation to the same or substantially the same facts. If the case examiners do reach such a decision, they should give reasons for any apparent inconsistency

- the case examiners are entitled to assess the weight of the evidence.
- the presence of an interim order or previous interim orders is not relevant to considering whether the "realistic prospect" test has been met. The test and considerations for the imposition of an interim order is different in many regards. The presence of an interim order therefore should not be a factor in considering whether to refer an allegation to the FTP Committee, as the presence of an interim order does not constitute a factual finding.

Warnings

Should the decision be made that the matter under consideration is not to be referred to the FTP Committee, case examiners may decide that the issue of a warning is appropriate. Reasons for the warning should be clear and the terms of any warning must not seek to impose on a registrant a more onerous obligation than that required under the terms of the current GOC Code or Standards. Any instruction as to future conduct must be qualified to indicate that the registrant must take "reasonable and proportionate steps" to comply with the relevant provisions of the Code, rather than seek to impose an absolute obligation to do so. In providing information Case examiners must avoid giving the impression that a finding or determination of matters of fact has been made on substantive issues arising from the complaint.

It should be considered that a warning issued by case examiners is a record of concern that, while not requiring referral to the FTP Committee, is potentially significant. Although not in legislation, warnings will currently remain for four years from the date of the warning letter and are not shown on the publicly available GOC Register but are recorded against the registrant's entry in the relevant register.

Taking no further action

If an allegation is considered as not needing to be referred to the FTP Committee or results in the issue of a warning no further action results.

The case examiners may decide to close a case without taking any further action when:

- the allegation demonstrates no issue that could call into question a registrant's fitness to practice
- the alleged facts, even if proved, are not serious enough to result in that registrant's fitness to practice being impaired to the extent that would justify action being taken against their registration, and a warning is deemed unnecessary
- the alleged facts, if proved, may demonstrate that a registrant's fitness to practice is impaired, but there is no realistic prospect of being able to prove the alleged facts for evidential reasons, and a warning is deemed unnecessary.

In these situation case examiners may decide to issue advice to a registrant — however such advice has no formal status, it is simply advice. Case examiners should draft the advice carefully so as to be clear that they are not issuing a warning. A warning is a formal response from the GOC to an allegation under Section 13D of the Opticians Act which is recorded against a registrant's entry in the register, whereas advice is an informal comment on the matter from the case examiners to assist the registrant.

How are decisions recorded?

All decisions made by case examiners are recorded in writing setting out full and detailed reasoning for the decision made. It is important to ensure reasoning is clear particularly in cases where for example:

- some but not all the factual particulars are being referred to the FTP Committee, or where more than one ground of impairment has been alleged, in order to be clear which factual particulars and allegations are being referred and on which ground of impairment
- numerous documents have been submitted to support the allegation; the decision should be clear that these have been read. The decision

should refer to specific document(s)/section(s) and set out how these relate to that part of the decision

- the case examiners agree that there is a realistic prospect of finding the factual particulars proved but decide not to refer the allegations due to evidence of insight and remediation. The case examiners should set out why the evidence is so compelling as to decide not to refer the allegation of impairment
- the decision of the case examiners, which will not have resolved disputes of fact, appears to discount the findings of an expert opinion.

Notification

Following the case examiners' decision, the complainant(s) and the registrant(s) concerned receive a letter from the GOC setting out the case examiners' decision and the reasons for that decision. In the case of individual registrants, their employer will be informed of the case examiners' decision, but they will not be provided with the full decision.

The GOC may be instructed in some cases to refer an allegation to the police if it appears to relate to the commission of a criminal offence (or to refer the allegation to another enforcement agency, as appropriate).

Referral of cases from case examiners to the Investigation Committee (IC)

It is expected that in the current system case examiners will be able to deal with the majority of cases, however, there are two situations where cases must be referred to the Investigation Committee by the case examiners:

Situation 1

Where the case examiners decide that they require further information about a registrant's health and/or the standard or quality of their work before they can reach a decision on the case, they must refer the matter to the Investigating Committee, requesting that an assessor (or assessors) be appointed, and an assessment (or assessments) be directed. The IC may direct that any one or more of the following investigative actions should be carried out (including if required, more than one assessment):

- a health assessment of the individual registrant
- a performance assessment of the individual registrant

In these circumstances the IC must specify the matters on which the registrant is to be assessed.

If more than one assessor is appointed in respect of a performance assessment, the assessors must together prepare a joint report for the IC. In respect of a health assessment, each assessor will prepare a report. The registrant will be sent a copy of all reports prepared and may submit comments on the report(s) to the Registrar within 28 days of receipt.

Where a registrant co-operates and an assessment (or assessments) has taken place, the IC must refer the allegation back to the original case examiners. The case examiners will receive a copy of the assessment report (or reports), together with any information provided by the registrant. The case examiners then will resume their consideration of the matter. If a registrant fails to co-operate with, or submit to, an assessment (or assessments), the IC itself will proceed to consideration of the allegation. In these circumstances, the case examiners will cease to have any further involvement in the case.

Situation 2

Where the case examiners are not unanimous in their decision about the appropriate disposal of the matter i.e., they are unable to reach a unanimous decision in a particular case, they must inform the Registrar and the Registrar will refer the matter to the IC for them to determine how to dispose of the case.

What is the composition of the Investigation Committee and how does it work?

The membership of the IC and its decision-making procedures are laid down in The General Optical Council (Committee Constitution) Rules

2005 SI 1474 and The General Optical Council (Committee Constitution) (Amendment) Rules Order of Council 2008 SI 3113. Currently the IC has a total of nine members and is a mixture of lay and professional members. As laid down three members must be registered optometrists, two must be registered dispensing opticians, three must be lay persons, and one must be a medical practitioner.

To be quorate and make decisions about an allegation a minimum of five IC members must be present and this must include at least one optometrist, one dispensing optician and one lay member. The IC meets in private and is able to obtain independent legal advice. The complainant, registrant and their representatives are not allowed to attend IC meetings. The IC takes its decisions by a simple majority vote (the Chair does not have a casting vote). No Committee member may abstain from voting and where the votes cast are equal, the legislation states that the Committee must decide in favour of the registrant. The GOC published Guidance for the IC in 2017.

As with case examiners at any stage, prior to making their final decision, the IC may adjourn their consideration of a case pending further investigation and inform the Registrar who will undertake the further investigation. The Registrar will provide any additional evidence obtained to the registrant and, where appropriate, to the maker of the allegation, giving them a reasonable opportunity to respond. The Registrar will then provide the IC with all additional evidence, together with any further comments and the IC will resume its consideration of the matter.

If, during the course of considering the allegations, the IC considers that there may be evidence (either from the complaint made to the GOC or from any further investigation) of allegations not included by the Registrar, or that the allegations should be amended, the IC should adjourn its consideration of the case and inform the Registrar. The Registrar may then consider the matters raised and determine whether additional or alternative allegations should be drafted and after the registrant has had an opportunity to respond to any new or amended allegations/evidence (Rule 12), the IC would resume its consideration of the matter.

Decision-making process

The whole investigation process must be transparent and when making any decision about a particular allegation, the IC will consider not only the original allegation and any evidence that has been gathered by the GOC, but also any written representations that have been received from the registrant concerned. The rules state that a registrant must be given copies of any information or documents received in support of the allegation and allowed 28 days in which to make any written representations before the IC considers the allegation(s).

The IC also will consider any comments received from the complainant, made once the complainant has seen any written representations made by the registrant. Any comments from the complainant are also copied to the registrant.

The IC must not be influenced by the type, or volume, of evidence that has been gathered by the GOC, except where that evidence is relevant to their consideration of a particular allegation. In wider terms, the overall volume of evidence gathered is only relevant to the decision-making process if the IC agree that it is insufficient for them to reach a decision and that they need to adjourn their consideration pending further details. The volume/type of evidence, in isolation, is not relevant to whether an allegation is likely to pass the realistic prospect test.

There may be cases that involve concerns about several aspects of a registrant's fitness to practise. In making a decision, it is the cumulative effect of all impairing factors that must be taken into account. Health and performance assessments are part of the process of collecting evidence (for individual registrants), but there may also be other evidence that the IC will need to consider when reaching a decision. Where the factual particulars relate to several aspects of a registrant's fitness to practise, the IC should include in its decision references to any specific representations or evidence it has considered in reaching its decision.

Where the IC's decision discounts, either fully or partially, an undisputed expert opinion, it must provide very clear reasons for this. The IC must also remember that as with the case examiners its role is not to make decisions on the facts, but only to determine whether the facts support a FTP referral.

What are the potential outcomes of an IC review?

The IC has four options available:

(1) refer the case to the FTP Committee;
(2) issue a warning;
(3) invite the registrant to undergo a voluntary performance review; or
(4) take no further action.

If the case is escalated upwards to the FTP Committee, the IC has the additional responsibility of deciding whether an interim order should be considered while the case was investigated.

What are Interim orders?

The need for an interim order hearing arises where either the Registrar or a case examiner considers an allegation serious enough to put the public at risk. The Registrar will refer the matter to the FTP Committee for consideration and notify the involved parties. An interim Order Hearing is not a full hearing, and the evidence is not tested to the same level, and this is to enable the Committee to provide a speedy consideration not of the case itself but of the possible risk that the allegation poses for the public.
An interim order can result in:

• suspension of a registrant completely
• temporary removal of an entry relating to a specialty or proficiency
• registration being subject to conditions or compliance with requirements imposed by the FTP Committee.

Normally an Interim Order can last for a maximum of 18 months, unless extended by the relevant court, and will be subject to regular reviews during that period. Such orders have a direct and rapid impact on a registrant and therefore should only be made where the FTP Committee are satisfied that it is necessary for the protection of members of the public; or otherwise in the public interest; or in the interests of a registrant.

Notification of an application for an interim order

Where a matter has been referred to the FTP Committee to consider the making of an interim order, the Registrar must serve on the registrant a Notice of Interim Order. This notice would state the date, time and venue of the interim order hearing and include a statement setting out the alleged facts constituting the basis of the application and enclose copies of any supporting documentary evidence. The registrant should be informed of their right to attend the hearing and be represented and of the power of the Fitness to Practise Committee to proceed in the registrant's absence. The registrant is required to inform the Registrar by a specified date whether they intend to do all or any of the following:

- attend the hearing,
- oppose the making of the interim order,
- be represented at the hearing.

Unless the Registrar is of the view that the public interest requires earlier action, the interim order hearing must take place no earlier than 7 days after the date upon which the Notice of Interim Order Hearing was sent to the registrant. Where the date, time or venue is varied for any reason the Registrar must take such efforts as are reasonable in the circumstances to inform the registrant of the variations before the interim order hearing.

How are interim order hearings conducted?

Interim order hearings are private hearings at which the FTP Committee may receive any evidence which appears to it to be fair and relevant to its consideration. However as mentioned above an interim hearing is not a full hearing to determine the case but to decide on risk and normally oral evidence would only be given where the FTP Committee considered it desirable to enable the Committee to reach a decision. Presentation of additional written evidence by a party may be allowed by the FTP Committee where the registrant consents or after consultation with the legal adviser but only if the Committee is satisfied that it would aid the hearing. In these circumstances the additional written evidence may be taken even though a copy has not been provided to the other party in advance of the hearing, or where the author is not being called as a witness.

According to The General Optical Council (Fitness to Practise) Rules Order of Council 2013 (SI 2013:2537) unless the Fitness to Practise Committee otherwise decides, the normal order of proceedings is as follows:

- The Presenting Officer informs the Committee of the reasons why it may be necessary to make an interim order against the registrant and provides any relevant evidence
- The registrant responds by demonstrating why they consider an interim order should not be made and may present any relevant evidence;
- Having heard both representation the Committee must deliberate in private remembering that at this stage this is not a determination of fact but on an interim order
- Once a decision has been made the Committee must announce in public its decision, together with the reasons for reaching that decision.

What is involved in fitness to practise hearings?

General considerations

The purpose of these hearing panels, following an IC referral, is to review all the facts and to take relevant evidence to determine if the alleged facts are proven. Once this has been completed if the facts are found proven the committee must consider whether the facts indicate that the registrant's fitness to practice by virtue of the decision on facts is impaired. Should the committee decide that fitness to practice is indeed impaired then a decision on the appropriate sanctions to be put in place has to be made and mitigating factors may be considered at this final stage.

Representation

The parties to hearings before the FTP Committee are entitled to be heard and if not representing themselves may be represented by:

- a person with a general qualification (within the meaning of section 71 of the Courts and Legal Services Act 1990(**a**));
- an advocate in Scotland, or a solicitor entitled to appear in the Court of Session and the High Court of Justiciary;
- a member of the Bar of Northern Ireland or Solicitor of the Supreme Court of Northern Ireland.

In addition to the persons mentioned above a registrant may be represented by a representative of any professional organisation of which the registrant is a member or where the registrant is a business registrant, a responsible officer of the body corporate or if the registrant requests and the Fitness to Practise Committee agrees, any other person.

Where an individual registrant is not represented as outlined above but chooses to self- represent, they may be accompanied and advised by any person, but that person is not entitled to address the Committee without its permission.

The exception is that a person who gives evidence at a hearing is not, without the permission of the Fitness to Practise Committee, entitled to represent or accompany the registrant at the hearing.

Proceeding in the absence of a registrant

Where a registrant is neither present nor represented at a hearing, the Fitness to Practise Committee may nevertheless proceed if it is satisfied that all reasonable efforts have been made to notify the registrant of the hearing and having taken account of any reason for absence provided by the registrant it is satisfied that it is in the public interest to proceed.

Hearings in public

Substantive hearings before the Fitness to Practise Committee must be held in public. However, in the following situations and where the FTP Committee consider it appropriate having looked at all the circumstances, including the public interest, proceedings or parts of proceedings may be heard in private when considered:

- in the interests of the maker of an allegation (where one has been made)
- in the interests of any patient or witness concerned
- in the interests of the registrant;

The exception is that in the situation where the Fitness to Practise Committee is considering the physical or mental health of a registrant it would be a private hearing.

Where an allegation has been received by the GOC falling outside any of the above procedures it will result in what is called a procedural or substantive hearing. These are held in private and designed for both parties to agree dates for exchanging witness and expert evidence and for setting a proposed date for the substantive hearing. The hearings are conducted by two lay members and one professional member of the hearings panel, plus one legal adviser. Deadlines are set in legislation to determine the point by which evidence and hearing bundles must have been prepared and shared by the parties involved.

Substantive Hearing

A substantive hearing normally takes place at least 28 days after the procedural hearing although provided both parties agree to it, a substantive hearing may occasionally follow on directly from a procedural hearing. These hearings are conducted by three lay and two professional members of the hearings panel, plus one legal adviser. One of the Lay members will take the role of Chair. The substantive hearing decides on the validity of the allegation and any actions required. The decision on the validity of the allegation is based on the same burden of proof as in a civil action i.e. on the balance of probabilities and it is for the GOC to prove that the allegation is valid.

Who may be used as an Adviser in hearings?

There are three types of advisers that may be involved with the FTP process:

Legal advisers

A legal adviser must be present at all hearings to advise the committee. The advice given should cover any matters of law, evidence or procedure which are referred to the legal adviser by the Committee. In addition, the legal adviser can offer advice when it appears to the legal adviser that, without intervention, there is the possibility of a mistake of law being made or the legal adviser becomes aware of any irregularity in the conduct of the proceedings. Advice is also available on the drafting of the FTP committee's decisions.

It is also the role of the Legal adviser to ensure that any advice given on matters of law, evidence or procedure are shared with all parties.

Clinical advisers

Where a registrant's physical or mental health is to be considered by the Fitness to Practise Committee a clinical adviser must be present at the hearing to offer specific advice to the Committee on the significance of any evidence presented that relates to the registrant's physical or mental health. As with legal advice to the committee such advice must be shared with all parties.

Specialist advisers

Where a specialist adviser has been appointed in relation to a matter to be considered at a substantive hearing, the adviser must be present at the hearing and advise the FTP Committee on matters relating to the specialty for which they have been appointed. Once again it is a requirement that any advice given is shared by all parties.

What is the order of proceedings at substantive hearings?

There is a set procedure for substantive hearings and unless there are particular reasons to vary this as determined by a FTP committee the hearing will proceed along the legislated lines. The Chair of the panel requires the registrant's name and registration number to be confirmed by the registrant or if the registrant is not present confirmed by the Presenting Officer and the Committee will hear and consider any preliminary legal arguments.

The allegation against the registrant is read by the Hearings Manager and the Chair checks whether the registrant wishes to make any admissions in relation to the allegation. Where facts are admitted the Chair must announce that such facts have been found proved but where facts remain in dispute, the Presenting Officer opens the case for the Council and may cite evidence and call witnesses in support of it.

Before opening their case the registrant (or their representative) may question whether sufficient evidence has been cited to enable the disputed facts to be found proved or even if the facts were likely proved they would support a finding of impairment. The Fitness to Practise Committee must then consider the statement by the registrant and make a decision as to whether sufficient evidence has been put forward in which case the hearing would proceed, and the registrant may cite evidence and call witnesses in support of their evidence.

The Committee are able during the course of these submissions to ask any questions of fact to clarify information that has been presented and having heard both parties must then consider and announce its findings of fact giving reasons for the decision. The Fitness to Practise Committee then may receive further evidence and hear any further submissions from the parties as to whether, based on any facts found proved, the alleged grounds of impairment are established. Having considered any further evidence or submissions if the Committee conclude that the alleged grounds of impairment are established it announces that fact and provides its reasons for the decision.

Only at this stage is consideration given to whether the registrant's fitness to practise is impaired and if it decides that it is then the Committee will hear further submissions in relation to the appropriate sanctions that should be imposed. At any stage before making its decision as to the imposition of a sanction or warning, the Fitness to Practise Committee may adjourn for further information or reports to be obtained to assist it in exercising its functions. Once determined the Committee announce its decision as to the sanction or warning (if any) to be imposed, giving reasons for the decision.

Decisions of the Fitness to Practise Committee are to be taken by a simple majority and no member of a Committee may abstain from voting. Should a situation arise where the votes are equal the issue will be decided in favour of the registrant.

What is impairment?

A registrant's fitness to practise may be impaired only on certain grounds as outlined earlier and these are set out at Section 13D (2) and (3) of the Opticians Act 1989. Those grounds vary, depending on whether it is a business registrant, a student registrant, or an individual practitioner. To assist with decision making case law has established the following principles regarding the concepts of "misconduct" and "deficient professional performance":

- "misconduct" does not mean any type of breach of the duty owed by a business registrant or an individual registrant to their patient, it relates to a serious breach which indicates that the business registrant's or an individual registrant's fitness to practise is impaired. Negligence does not necessarily constitute "misconduct" but negligent acts or omissions which are particularly serious may amount to "misconduct". In these circumstances a single negligent act or omission is less likely to cross the threshold of "misconduct" than multiple acts or omission. However, there may be some circumstances in which a single negligent act or omission, if particularly serious, could be characterised as "misconduct".

- "deficient professional performance" indicates a standard of performance which is unacceptably low. A single instance of negligent treatment would be unlikely to constitute "deficient professional performance" although if serious enough it may. Therefore, unless there are exceptional circumstances, "deficient professional performance" should be based on consideration of a fair sample of work. There is however no definition of "fair".

How are decisions made?

After deliberation in private, decisions of Fitness to Practise panels are taken by a simple majority vote. As part of that process no Chair of a Committee may exercise a casting vote and no member of a Committee may abstain from voting.

In rare circumstances where the panel for exceptional reasons is not made up of an odd number of members if the votes are equal then the Committee decision must be taken as deciding that the issue under consideration is in favour of the registrant.

What sanctions are available to an FTP panel?

Erasure from the registers

If this decision is made the outcome is that the registrant cannot practise as an optometrist/dispensing optician, or in the case of a student registrant, cannot continue with their training and the registrant's name is erased from the relevant register(s). If the erasure relates only to a specialty register the individual's name is removed from the specific specialty register and they cannot perform any duties associated with that specialty.

This sanction cannot be imposed if a registrant's fitness to practise is found to be impaired because of adverse physical and/or mental health.

Suspension from the register

Where a registrant is suspended their name is temporarily removed from the relevant register(s). The registrant cannot practise as an optometrist/

dispensing optician, or in the case of a student registrant, cannot continue with their training for the duration of the suspension.

If the suspension relates to a specialty register, the registrant may not perform any duties associated with that specialty for the duration of the suspension. The maximum suspension period is 12 months.

Once the suspension period has ended, a review hearing is held to determine whether the registrant should have the suspension lifted, remain suspended, or if other sanctions should be imposed.

Conditional registration

In this situation, specific conditions are set to restrict the way that a registrant can work, and the registrant remains on the relevant register providing the conditions are being met. Conditions are individual and may for example relate to specific groups of patients that should not be seen, a level of supervision or a requirement to undertaking additional training.

Once the period of conditional registration has ended, a review hearing is held to determine whether the conditions should be lifted, the registrant should remain subject to conditions, or if other sanctions should be imposed.

Financial penalty

If considered appropriate by the FTP panel a financial penalty of no more than £50,000 can be imposed on a registrant. The penalty must be paid within a specified length of time which is set by the committee. If the penalty is not paid, the GOC may take court action to recover the full amount. In the case of a registrant's failure to pay the fine the issue is reported to the Investigation Committee for further action.

Warning

Even in situations where the hearings panel decide that a registrant's fitness to practise is **not** impaired, but it is felt that there is an issue with the performance they still may issue the registrant with a warning about their future conduct or performance.

What are review hearings?

This type of hearing takes place following a panel decision where the following milestones are reached:

- within the first six months of an interim suspension order, and every six months thereafter for as long as the registrant is suspended from the register
- at the end of a registrant's suspension period, if a substantive hearing has not yet taken place. The panel will decide if new sanctions should be imposed on the registrant, if the current sanction is adequate, or if all sanctions should be lifted
- at the end of a conditional registration period. The panel will decide if new sanctions should be imposed on the registrant, if the current sanction is adequate, or if all sanctions should be lifted.

The panel for these hearings is composed of two lay members and one professional member for interim order reviews or three lay members and two professional members of the independent hearings panel for all other review hearings, plus one legal adviser.

Registration appeal/application for restoration hearing

A registration appeal hearing is held if an individual is refused entry to the register, and they wish to appeal against the Registrar's decision. A restoration application hearing is held when a practitioner has been erased from the register for disciplinary reasons and wishes to apply to re-join the register.

The panel for this type of hearing is composed of three lay and two professional members of the "Registration Appeals Committee".

How are hearings reported?

A verbatim record, in either written or electronic form, must be taken of every hearing before the Fitness to Practise Committee. A copy of this record is available on request from the GOC. The outcomes of all hearings are reported on the GOC website as is the timetable for hearings.

Can costs and expenses be awarded?

The Fitness to Practise Committee may, as it thinks fit, summarily assess the costs of any party to a substantive hearing or to any review hearing other than a hearing to review an interim order and may order any party to pay all or part of the costs or expenses of any other party relating to that hearing.

Chapter 14

Regulation Relating to the Use of Drugs

The use of drugs by the optometry profession has gone through a roller-coaster series of changes culminating in the introduction of independent prescribing rights in 2008 enabling access to a much wider range of drugs for those practitioners with the additional qualification. To understand the position of the use of drugs by optometrists however requires a review of the fundamental regulation the Medicines Act of 1968 that formalized medicine regulation and set the basis for supply and use of pharmaceutical and other related products in the UK and is still current in the UK.

Actioning the Medicines Act 1968

In January 1978, the Government published the long-awaited statutory instruments bringing into force Part Ill of the Medicines Act 1968 and announced that the "appointed day" would be 1 February 1978. Such was the extent and complexity of the changes made in these Orders that a supplementary Order had to be made later, postponing certain of the provisions for 6 months. This delay was to give the pharmaceutical industry and the profession of pharmacy sufficient time to come to terms with the new regulations concerning the sale and supply of some drugs.

Not least to be affected by the complex new regulations was the optometrist, who gained the right to supply, as well as use, a greater range of drugs than before. To understand the development of the provisions relating to the use of drugs by optometrists, it is necessary first briefly to summarize the various parts of the Medicines Act 1968 and then look at the subsequent Orders made.

The Medicines Act 1968, covering as it does such a wide range of activities concerned with the production and supply of medicines, was no mean document and was divided into eight parts, containing in all 136 sections and eight schedules. Schedules 5-8 listed all the previous enactments to be repealed or amended with the coming into force of the main Act.

Part I of the Medicines Act 1968 deals with administration; s.2 sets up the Medicines Commission and Committees under it. The Medicines Commission consisted of not fewer than eight members, representing the following "activities" — medicine, veterinary medicine, pharmacy, pharmaceutical industry, and chemistry.

The 45 sections of Part II deal with the licensing of the manufacture, import, export, and wholesale of medicinal products. No person may manufacture or assemble or wholesale any product without a licence to do so. Such a "blanket" law was, of course, subject to many exemptions. For example, it would be time consuming for a pharmacist to obtain a licence every time a particular prescription was to be made for a particular patient and this activity was thus exempted from the need to obtain a license for manufacture under these conditions. There were further exemptions for doctors, dentists, veterinary practitioners, nurses, and midwives. There were also exemptions for herbal remedies and there were transitional exemptions for products which were on the market on the appointed day.

The most important sections as far as the optometrist is concerned were included in Part III, which deals with the sale or supply of medicinal products. To understand the implications of the various Orders introduced in February 1978 it is necessary to look at specific sections of this Part of the Act in detail.

Section 51 allowed the Minister to set up a "General Sale List" of drugs which could be reasonably sold without the supervision of a pharmacist. Section 53 allowed for certain drugs to be sold by automatic machine (i.e., an automatic machine section to the General Sale List). All drugs not on this "General Sale List" may be sold only by "a person lawfully conducting a retail pharmacy business" or on premises registered as a pharmacy and under the supervision of a pharmacist (s.52). This restriction previously was applied by including a substance in Part I of the Poisons List, when sale could be made only by an "authorized seller of poisons" (note the change in title). Now, paradoxically, it became the non-inclusion of a substance in a list that brought this restriction into force. Since it allowed certain exempt substances to be sold other than at a pharmacy even if they were not included on a General Sale List, a very important rider to the regulation stated: "*subject to any exemption conferred by or under this part of the Act*". This rider was included in section 52 and several other sections of the Act.

Sections 53 and 54 lay down the conditions under which General Sale List substances may be sold, and ss.55–57 lay down broad exemptions from s.52.

Further restrictions were imposed under s.58 that allowed for another list of medicinal substances called the "Prescription Only List" to be set up. Under subsection (2), medicines on the Prescription Only List could be supplied only in accordance with a prescription issued by an "appropriate practitioner" (a term defined in subsection (1) as being doctors, dentists, or veterinarians). The remainder of s.58 dealt with exemptions from this restriction, subject to conditions that may be defined in the relevant Orders.

The rest of Part III dealt with other conditions concerning the sale or supply of medicinal substances and as not relevant to optometry are not discussed here.

The remaining Parts IV, V, VI, VII and VIII of the Act related to pharmacies, containers, promotion of sales, official publications, and miscellaneous provisions respectively.

Nowhere in the Act were specific medicinal substances listed. The inclusion of substances in the General Sale List or in the Prescription Only List was the subject of the various Orders brought into effect on 1 February 1978 and subsequently revised.

General Sale List

The General Sale List is a list of human and veterinary drugs defined by s. 51 of the Medicines Act and contains the common (and some not so common) medicinal substances which can be sold other than at a pharmacy. Provided that s.53 is complied with, an optometrist may sell any substance on the General Sale List.

Schedule 6 of the Medicines (General Sale List) Order (SI 1977/2129) however, lists medicinal products that are not on the General Sale List and includes products marketed as medicinal eye drops or eye ointments. Thus, all medicinal eye drops, whether for human or for animal use, were not on general sale even though the active principle may have been included in the list.

Prescription Only Medicines (POM) List

Many of the drugs commonly in use by optometrists were included in Schedule 1 of the POM List. Even though the schedule exempted many of these drugs from the class of prescription only when they were applied externally, local ophthalmic use was often excluded from the exemption. For example, atropine was prescription only unless applied externally by a route other than to the eye.

Eye drops and eye ointment were singled out in regulation for special attention both by their exclusion from the General Sale List (GSL) and in the external application exemption from the POM list.

Pharmacy List

This was a "catch all" list and any preparation that did not appear on the GSL or the POM lists was automatically covered by the Pharmacy (P) list as defined by section 52 of the Medicines Act. All drugs included on this list would normally be sold or supplied from a registered pharmacy under the supervision of a registered pharmacist. In the case of a P medicine that is an eye-drop or ointment it could be used and supplied by an optometrist — supply being by way of a signed order for presentation to a pharmacist.   •

Effect on Optometry

The complexity of the regulation is demonstrated by the regulation covering supply by an optometrist. Initially published under the terms of the

Medicines (Prescription only) Order 1977/Number 2127 and amended by The Medicines (Prescription only) Order Amendment Number 2 1978/ Number 287, Schedule 4 Part I 5(2), further revised by SI 1983/1212 and again by SI 1989/1852, as Schedule 3(1) 5 and 6 and by SI1997/1830 Schedule 5 part 1 is a list of exemptions from s.58(2) — the section by which a prescription is required before drugs on the list can be supplied. Paragraph 5 allowed pharmacists to supply certain specified eye drops or ointments subject to the presentation of an order signed by a registered optometrist. Paragraph 6 allowed optometrists to supply the same drugs in the course of their professional practice or in an emergency. Interestingly this schedule only gave exemption from s.58, it does not give exemption from s.52 (supply only by a pharmacist). The exemption from this latter section was given in another separate order — the Medicines (Pharmacy and General Sale — Exemption) Order 1977 as amended by SI 1978/ Number 988, and SI 1980/1924 — which exempted optometrists from the requirements of s.52 for the same drugs in the schedule. This Order also provided a general, transitional exemption from s.52 for products that could have been supplied lawfully before the appointed day. This exemption lasted for 2 years.

One further order, the Medicines (Sale or Supply) (Miscellaneous Provisions) Regulations 1977, SI 1977/2132, as amended by SI 1978/989 and subsequently included in SI 1980/1923, allowed the optometrist to obtain and use a further range of drugs. The regulation related to wholesale dealing, which is defined in the Medicines Act 1968 as being "supply to a person for retail sale, or for administering to a human being in the course of a business carried on by him". Since this Order did not give exemption from s.52, only the latter purpose was catered for, i.e., optometrists may use these drugs in their practice but must not supply them to their patients. Most of the drugs in this Order were the local anaesthetics that would never be given to patients for their own use. Details of individual drugs listed at the time were to be found in "The Optometrists Formulary" published by the College of Optometrists in 1998 and regularly updated.

In specific emergency circumstances, optometrists may decide that the best course of action for the patient was to supply them directly with exempted prescription only medicines or ophthalmic pharmacy only medicinal products. In such a case, the optometrist may re-label pre-packed preparations without holding a licence for assembly. This position had been achieved through the GOC's application for a general exemption for registered opticians under the requirements of Article 2 of the Medicines (Exemptions from Licences) (Assembly) order 1979 Number 114. The exemption did not apply to contact lens fluids and a separate individual exemption would be needed for this situation under the requirements of Medicines (Contact Lens Fluids and Other Substances) (Exemption from Licences) Order 1979 Number 1585.

If re-labelling was undertaken by the optometrist, then to meet the labelling regulations for a dispensed medicinal product, the following information, written in indelible ink, was required on the product:

- The name of the patient.
- The directions for use.
- The words "Keep out of reach of children".
- The phrase "For external use only".
- The date of supply.
- The name and address of the supplying optometrist.

Although the Medicines Act 1968 was wide ranging in its effects, it is not the only Act that affected the sale and supply of drugs. So-called "controlled drugs" were covered by the Misuse of Drugs Act 1971. All standard eye preparations of cocaine came under this Act and hence could not be used by an optometrist.

Contact lens care products underwent a change in 1995. Prior to this date they were required to have a product license from the Medicines Control Agency (this became in 2003 the Medicines and Healthcare products Regulatory Agency (MHRA)). Subsequent to this date all contact lens care products were required to have a CE marking and number. Should an optometrist wish to re-label a contact lens care product the Medical Devices Agency would be able to provide the appropriate information and licensing.

The effect of the legislation was to increase the range of drugs that the optometrist may use and supply. Apart from in an emergency, the use or supply of drugs had to be in line with the practice of the profession of optometry as defined in the Opticians Act 1989 or laid down by the GOC. Nothing in the 1968 Act changed the restrictions concerning treatment of adverse ocular conditions.

As mentioned earlier The Medicines Act is still in force today and continues to be amended and updated as required by Statutory Instrument.

Medicines and Healthcare products Regulatory Agency (MHRA)

The MHRA was mentioned above and is an executive agency of the Department of Health and Social Care responsible for ensuring that medicines and medical devices meet safety standards and are effective. The Agency was formed in 2003 with the merger of the Medicines Control Agency (MCA) and the Medical Devices Agency (MDA). In terms of the Medicines Act and optometry the MHRA are responsible for determining the range of drugs available to optometrists for use in practice and provide a list on the Agency website — this list as of January 2022 is under review and shown below.

MHRA are also responsible for the Medical Devices Regulations, and this is applied to optics through glazing of spectacle frames that is classed as assembly and the surfacing of spectacle lenses that is classed as manufacturing. Practices receiving remotely edged lenses and fitting them into a frame on site for example also require registration with MHRA as this process is considered to be assembly. This means that businesses undertaking these tasks, including practices which assemble or glaze spectacles, must be registered using form RG2. Similarly, any supplier of an own brand medical device (e.g., spectacle frames) must be registered with MHRA using form RG2.

The Crown Report

Following on from the publication of the Department of Health's white paper "Primary Care: Delivering the Future" (1996) a group was established in 1997 to undertake a "Review of Prescribing, Supply and Administration of Medicines".

The aims of the group were to:

- Develop a framework to determine the circumstances in which health professionals could undertake new roles regarding the prescribing, supply, and administration of medicines
- Consider the implications for legislation and professional training

The identified constraints for change were identified as:

- Any changes to existing roles must at the very least maintain, and preferably enhance, patient safety
- Changes needed to be cost effective
- There should be demonstrable benefits to patient care

An interim report from the team "Review of Prescribing, supply and administration of medicines — a report on the supply and administration of medicines under Group Protocols" was published in 1998 and the Final report in 1999.

The outcome of the final report was a series of recommendations to take forward prescribing of medicines. Two new classes of prescriber were suggested:

o Independent who would assess patients with undiagnosed conditions, make a diagnosis and be responsible for decisions about the clinical management required including prescribing
o Dependent who would be responsible for the continuing care of a patient who had been assessed by an independent prescriber

Optometrists appeared in the list of professions recommended for inclusion as independent prescribers. The report states *"Optometrists' expertise relating to the eye and visual system, coupled with the use of specialised diagnostic instruments, is the basis of the care they provide in the community, including domiciliary visits. Having established a diagnosis, prescribing would allow them to provide effective treatment for emergency eye conditions and non-sight threatening eye conditions."*

The developing framework for use of drugs in optometry

Around the same time as the Crown report was released the GOC in 2000 changed the rules relating to injury or disease formally allowing optometrists to decide not to refer a patient with an ocular abnormality to a medical practitioner but instead to render appropriate therapeutic treatment. An issue at this time however was that the range of therapeutic agents available to optometrists was restricted and therefore the range of conditions that could be managed was also restricted. This situation was partially improved by changes to regulation in 2005 that updated the range of agents available, relaxed the emergency clause for use of P and GSL agents and recognised supplementary prescribing by optometrists. This raft of Statutory instruments changed the way that optometry could work (*The Medicines (Pharmacy and General Sale — Exemption) Amendment Order 2005 SI2005 766, The Medicines for Human Use (Prescribing) (Miscellaneous Amendments) Order SI2005 1507, The Medicines (Sale or Supply) (Miscellaneous Amendments) Regulations 2005 SI2005 1520, The Medicines for Human Use (Prescribing) (Miscellaneous Amendments) (No 2) Order SI2005 3324).*

Signed orders

As part of the same exercise of change the POMs available to optometrists were identified as out of date with several of the drugs included no longer commercially available and the list was reviewed and updated. The POMs available to optometrists for supply could be sold or supplied directly to patients as part of practice and in emergency situations only. Supply was via a signed order which the patient could present to a registered pharmacist. Such an order should contain:

- *The optometrist's name and address*
- *The date*
- *The name and address of the patient*

- *The name of the drug*
- *Quantity, pharmaceutical form, and strength of the POM*
- *Labelling directions (where applicable)*
- *The original signature of the optometrist.*

The signed order must be written in indelible ink; this includes type-written and computer-generated orders. Although not a requirement the College of Optometrists recommend that the GOC number should be included on the order.

During this period of change there were "wins and losses" as far as optometry were concerned with the addition of some new agents but the removal of others that had been on the previous list of exemptions.

The relaxation of the law governing the supply of P and GSL medicines by optometrists allowed for the direct supply to a patient of any P medicine used in the course of an optometrist's professional practice such as lubricants, anti-allergy preparations and antimicrobials. The College at the time in its guidance stated:

> *"If they are supplying therapeutic drugs to their patients, practitioners have a duty to ensure that this drug is appropriate for the patient. This will mean the optometrist has to make a diagnosis of the patient's condition. Supply should normally only be made following an eye examination, or within a reasonable time afterwards. Patients should be made aware of the need to have their condition periodically reassessed to determine whether or not the drug is still appropriate. This is particularly important if the patient has already sought treatment elsewhere. All actions and advice should be noted on the patient record".*

Supplementary Prescribing for Optometrists

The Medicines (Sale or Supply) (Miscellaneous Amendments) Regulations 2005 (SI 2005 No. 1520) amended the Medicines for Human Use (Marketing Authorisations Etc) Regulations 1994 and the Medicines (Sale or Supply) (Miscellaneous Provisions) Regulations 1980 to extend supplementary prescribing to registered optometrists with approved training.

Supplementary prescribing is an arrangement whereby after a diagnosis by an independent prescriber, the supplementary prescriber can prescribe medicines as part of a Clinical Management Plan agreed with the independent prescriber for an individual patient. The plan sets out how much responsibility is to be delegated and refers to a named patient and their specific condition. Both the independent and supplementary prescriber must record their agreement to the plan before supplementary prescribing begins. Both prescribers must also share access to a common patient record.

Although there are no legal restrictions on the clinical conditions that a supplementary prescriber can treat, or the medicines they can prescribe (since this type of prescribing requires a prescribing partnership with an independent prescriber and an agreed clinical management plan before it can begin), it is most useful when dealing with long-term medical conditions.

To obtain specialist registration with the GOC as a supplementary prescriber involves a post registration course of further GOC approved training, followed by the College of Optometrists' Common Final Assessment (CFA) for specialist qualifications in therapeutics (supplementary prescribing). Supplementary prescribing was integrated into the CFA for independent prescribing in 2009.

Independent prescribing for optometrists

In August 2006, the Medicine and Healthcare Products Regulatory Agency (MHRA) and the Department of Heath held a public consultation on the introduction of independent prescribing (IP) for optometrists. Following the consultation, which was overwhelmingly supportive of the proposal, in June 2007 advice from the Commission for Human Medicines proposed to restrict the scope of optometrist IP (in line with nurse and pharmacist independent prescribers) by reference to the competence of the individual prescribing optometrist, rather than linking it to an approved formulary as it is for entry-level and Additional Supply (AS) prescribing. This meant that suitably qualified optometrists could prescribe any licensed medicine (except for controlled drugs or medicines for parenteral (injected) administration) for conditions affecting the eye, and the tissues surrounding the eye, within their recognised area of expertise and competence.

Legislation to achieve this was introduced by (The Medicines (Sale or Supply) (Miscellaneous Amendments) Regulations 2008). Further changes to the POM order came into effect in June 2008 (The Medicines for Human Use (Prescribing) (Miscellaneous Amendments) Order 2008) and the GOC began registration of optometrists with the required IP qualifications from 1st November 2009. The scope of optometrist independent prescribing is informed by the College of Optometrists' Clinical Management Guidelines (CMGs), which provide a source of evidence-based information on the diagnosis and management of several eye conditions that present in primary and first contact care. Independent prescribers can prescribe privately and, where suitable arrangements have been made, write an NHS prescription.

Since the changes the number of optometrists wishing to become independent prescribers has increased and the GOC has approved several university courses to offer postgraduate training to achieve the qualification and some are building the basic blocks for it into the undergraduate course. In addition to the training, accreditation for independent prescribing requires successful completion of the College of Optometrists' Common Final Assessment (CFA) for specialist qualifications in therapeutics (independent prescribing). One of the limiting factors initially to obtaining the qualification had been accessing suitable practical placements but changes to enable qualified optometry IPs to act as placement supervisors rather than ophthalmologists in HES has opened up this area.

Patient Group Directions

A mechanism by which optometrists were enabled to supply medicines that were not normally available to them was through Patient Group Directions. Legislation establishing PGDs was introduced in 2000 and the current legislation is included in The Human Medicines Regulations 2012 (see below). To support the use of PGDs guidance has been developed by the National Institute for Health and Care Excellence (NICE) and can be found at http://www.nice.org.uk/guidance/mpg2/resources.

Patient group directions (PGDs) are written instructions that enable specified health professionals including optometrists to supply or administer medicines to patients in planned circumstances. They take a significant amount of time and resource to develop and implement and can only be implemented if there is an advantage for the patient without compromising their safety. PGDs should be determined by a multi-disciplinary group including a doctor, a pharmacist and a representative of any professional group expected to supply the medicines under the PGD. It's good practice to involve local drug and therapeutics committees, area prescribing committees and similar advisory bodies. The expiry date for a PGD needs to be decided on a case-by-case basis in the interest of patient safety.

Arrangements need to be put in place for the security, storage and labelling of each medicine included on the PGD and the expiry date of the Direction should not be more than 3 years from the date the PGD was authorised. SI2012:1916 specifies that each PGD must contain specific information including:

- *The period during which the direction is to have effect.*
- *The description or class of medicinal product to which the direction relates.*
- *The clinical situations which medicinal products of that description or class may be used to treat or manage in any form.*
- *Whether there are any restrictions on the quantity of medicinal product that may be sold or supplied on any one occasion and, if so, what restrictions.*
- *The clinical criteria under which a person is to be eligible for treatment.*
- *Whether any class of person is excluded from treatment under the direction and, if so, what class of person.*
- *Whether there are circumstances in which further advice should be sought from a doctor or dentist and, if so, what circumstances.*
- *The pharmaceutical form or forms in which medicinal products of that description or class are to be administered.*

- *The strength, or maximum strength, at which medicinal products of that description or class are to be administered.*
- *The applicable dosage or maximum dosage.*
- *The route of administration.*
- *The frequency of administration.*
- *Any minimum or maximum period of administration applicable to medicinal products of that description or class.*
- *Whether there are any relevant warnings to note and, if so, what warnings.*
- *Whether there is any follow up action to be taken in any circumstances and, if so, what action and in what circumstances.*
- *Arrangements for referral for medical advice.*
- *Details of the records to be kept of the supply, or the administration, of products under the direction.*

Human Medicines Regulations 2012

In 2012 additional regulation introduced under the Medicines Act 1968 provided several important amendments (The Human Medicines Regulations SI 2012:1916). In this regulation medicinal product (in line with an EU definition) was defined as

- *any substance or combination of substances presented as having properties of preventing or treating disease in human beings; or*
- *any substance or combination of substances that may be used by or administered to human beings with a view to—*
  - *restoring, correcting or modifying a physiological function by exerting a pharmacological, immunological or metabolic action, or*
  - *making a medical diagnosis.*

Much of the regulation included here builds on the original 1968 Act and the main elements for optometrists relate to exemptions to the general requirements that are specified in Schedule 17. The need for exemptions is indicated by for example an inclusion in Part 2 to Schedule 1 of the SI dealing with classification of Medicinal products that states:

The following medicinal products shall be available only from a pharmacy — (a) a product comprising eye ointment.

The relevant optometry exemptions cover:

1. Exemption from restrictions on sale and supply of prescription only medicines under which registered optometrists can sell and supply a range of prescription only medicines in the course of their professional practice and which are not for parenteral (injection) administration. Chloramphenicol, tropicamide and cyclopentolate in specific forms and strengths are included here.

2. Exemptions from the restrictions in regulations for certain persons who sell, supply, or offer for sale or supply certain medicinal products. Optometrists can sell or supply under this exemption all medical products on a general sale list, all pharmacy medicines and prescription only medicines which are not for parenteral administration, and which are eye drops and are prescription only medicines due to the concentration of the active substance. The sale and supply however are still only available if used by an optometrist:
   - in the case of medicinal products on a general sale list and pharmacy medicines, in the course of their professional practice;
   - in the case of prescription only medicines, in the course of their professional practice and in an emergency.

3. Exemptions for those optometrists with an additional supply qualification registered with the GOC (see below).

What drugs can a registered optometrist use in practice?

Summing up the current position it is the type of registration with the GOC i.e., registered optometrist, additional supply optometrist or independent prescriber optometrist that determines drug access. Independent prescribers have access as described above to any licensed medicine (except for controlled drugs or medicines for parenteral (injected) administration) for conditions affecting the eye, and the tissues surrounding the eye, within their recognised area of expertise and competence. However, for the others the available drugs are regularly reviewed and listed and as of January 2022 a review of the list was underway. Access at that time according to the 2014 MHRA list under review is shown below.

Registered optometrists

Any registered optometrist is permitted to sell/ supply all GSL and P medicines. In an emergency a registered optometrist can also sell the following POMs as part of their professional practice that are not for administration by injection:

- eye drops that contain no more than 0.5% chloramphenicol
- eye ointments that contain no more than 1% chloramphenicol
- substances that contain:
  - o   cyclopentolate hydrochloride
  - o   fusidic acid
  - o   tropicamide

Pharmacies can sell or supply the above POMs to patients if a registered optometrist has given a valid signed order (see above for requirements).

Commonly used P medicines

All registered Optometrists are able to use P medicines containing:

- *antazoline (up to 1%)*
- *azelastine hydrochloride (up to 0.1% for the treatment of the signs and symptoms of allergic conjunctivitis)*
- *dibromopropamidine isethionate*
- *fluorescein sodium*
- *levocabastine (up to 0.05% for the symptomatic treatment of seasonal allergic conjunctivitis) (no longer available in ophthalmic preparations in the UK in 2021)*

- *lodoxamide (up to 0.1% for ocular signs and symptoms of allergic conjunctivitis)*
- *phenylephrine hydrochloride*
- *propamidine sethionate*
- *rose Bengal*
- *sodium cromoglicate (only for the treatment of acute seasonal allergic conjunctivitis or perennial allergic conjunctivitis and subject to a maximum strength of 2% for eye drops or 4% for eye ointment — products containing this substance are also subject to restrictions on maximum quantity, which may be sold or supplied as a P medicine and are not more than 10ml for eye drops and 5g for eye ointment)*
- *various tear supplements and ocular lubricants*
- *xylometazoline hydrochloride*

Additional supply optometrists

Additional supply optometrists accredited and registered with the General Optical Council can sell, supply, or write an order for an extended range of medicines in an emergency and as part of their professional practice that contains:

- *acetylcysteine*
- *atropine sulphate*
- *azelastine hydrochloride*
- *diclofenac sodium*
- *emedastine (no longer available in ophthalmic preparations in the UK in 2021)*
- *homatropine hydrobromide*
- *ketotifen*
- *levocabastine (no longer available in ophthalmic preparations in the UK in 2021)*
- *lodoxamide*
- *nedocromil sodium (no longer available in ophthalmic preparations in the UK in 2021)*
- *olopatadine*

- *pilocarpine hydrochloride*
- *pilocarpine nitrate*
- *polymyxin B/bacitracin*
- *polymyxin B/trimethoprim*
- *sodium cromoglycate*

A pharmacy can sell/ supply the above POMs if the order is signed by an additional supply optometrist. The list is under review as some of the listed items are no longer available and in other cases more effective treatments are available.

Wholesale supplies to registered optometrists

All registered optometrists can stock the exempted P and POM products and can obtain stocks of P medicines and some POMs to administer to their patients. These POMs are:

- *amethocaine hydrochloride*
- *lignocaine hydrochloride*
- *oxybuprocaine hydrochloride*
- *proxymetacaine hydrochloride*

An additional supply optometrist also can obtain thymoxamine hydrochloride if it becomes available.

Medicinal Products or Medical devices what's the difference?

In the UK the definition of a medicinal product has been adopted from Article 1 of European Directive 2001/83/EC as amended and shown below:

> *"Any substance or combination of substances presented as having properties for treating or preventing disease in human beings; [the first/ presentational limb]*

Any substance or combination of substances which may be used in, or administered to, human beings, either with a view to restoring, correcting or modifying physiological functions by exerting a pharmacological, immunological or metabolic action, or to making a medical diagnosis" [the second/functional limb]

Medicinal products may well fall under both limbs of the definition, but the European Court of Justice (ECJ) has confirmed that falling under either limb is sufficient to classify a product as a medicinal product (European Directive 2004/27/EC).

In 2002 UK regulation was introduced to cover a wide range of products that were considered as medical devices. According to the Medical Devices Regulations 2002 (SI 2002 No 618, as amended) a medical device is described as:

"Any instrument, apparatus, appliance, software, material or other article, whether used alone or in combination, together with any accessories, including the software intended by its manufacturer to be used specifically for diagnosis or therapeutic purposes or both and necessary for its proper application, which is intended by the manufacturer to be used for human beings for the purpose of:

- *diagnosis, prevention, monitoring, treatment or alleviation of disease*
- *diagnosis, monitoring, treatment, alleviation of or compensation for an injury or handicap*
- *investigation, replacement or modification of the anatomy or of a physiological process, or*
- *control of conception"*

Unlike a medicinal product, a medical device does not achieve its main intended action by pharmacological, immunological, or metabolic means although it can be assisted by these. The two definitions have a certain degree of flexibility and therefore overlap and hence some products are seen as "borderline" products. This creates problems for those products falling within both categories, but which are then defined as a medicinal product with restricted access.

Historically, the legislation on medicinal products predated medical device regulation (MDR) and so when regulation of medical devices came into force, some products transferred their regulatory control to MDR e.g., contact lens care products. As a result of changes to the definition of a medicinal product in European Directive 2004/27/EC, some categories previously regulated as medicines were now considered to be medical devices e.g., artificial tears. However, there are some apparent anomalies and for the optical professions the largest of these was the classification of fluorescein.

The problem with fluorescein arises as although it does not achieve its effect by pharmacological means it can be used for diagnostic purposes, under the EU definition therefore it was classified as a medicinal product rather than a medical device with restricted access. This makes it a P medicine regulated by the Medicines Act. Changes are being made to the regulations on borderline classification and the position of fluorescein should be clarified via this process.

In practical terms it is the use of fluorescein in the fitting of contact lenses that has been the main stumbling block as defining fluorescein as a medicinal product restricts access for certain groups. The UK situation has evolved following publication of a joint document from the professional bodies in 2013: *Clinical consensus panel report on the use of fluorescein in primary care* and while the European position is resolving no change to the original classification situation has been implemented in the UK. Latest information from the review in Europe in late 2021 appeared to offer a compromise by classifying fluorescein as either a medicinal product or a medical device dependent upon the usage specified in the product labelling.

Clinical Management Guidelines

Guidance on the use of drugs for specific conditions is available through *"The College of Optometrists Clinical Management Guidelines"*. The guidelines provide details of some of the more common conditions met by optometrists in routine practice and in addition to providing useful information on the condition and its differential diagnosis also provide information on both pharmacological and non-pharmacological management.

The College of Optometrists has produced a very helpful *Optometrists' Formulary* available on the College website to College members. The Formulary provides details on ophthalmic preparations such as:

- Legal classification
- Available preparations
- Drug type
- Classification
- Indications
- Contraindications
- Cautions
- Interactions
- Ocular side effects
- General side effects
- Dose
- Storage

As the regulatory situation is reviewed and modified at regular intervals and the range of drugs that are produced changes over time it is essential that all optometrists keep themselves updated as to what is available for their use in practise.

Adverse Drug Reactions (ADRs) Reporting scheme

The purpose of this scheme is to provide an early warning that the safety of a medicine or a medical device may require further investigation. The Yellow Card Scheme is an integral part of monitoring. Developed in 1964, it is the UK system for collecting information on suspected adverse drug interactions. Originally just for doctors, it was extended in the late 1990s and is now open to all including members of the public. It is important for practitioners to report problems experienced by their patients with medicines or medical devices as these are used to identify issues which might not have been previously known about.

All suspected adverse drug reactions (ADRs) should be reported using the MHRA Yellow Card system — the name is there as the initial scheme used yellow postcards. A Yellow card is a standard form used to report a suspected ADR that can be submitted online via the MHRA website at yellowcard.mhra.gov.uk or by post or by using the appropriate app. The scheme also covers the reporting of adverse incidents to herbal or homeopathic remedies and to Medical Devices.

Chapter 15

Ethics and Guidance within the Profession

General Background

Before 1988, there were two major sources of ethical and professional guidance; the one produced by the professional body the British College of Optometrists (BCO) and the other (N22), in support of its regulations, by the statutory body the General Optical Council (GOC). Notice N22 however, published by the GOC in March 1987 was after much discussion withdrawn in 1988 and the decision made by the GOC at that stage that for future cases in which professional conduct was under review a 'peer group' view would be used.

GOC guidance

Under the Opticians Act 1989, the GOC was required to issue guidance to registrants in relation to their fitness to practise, fitness to undertake training, and fitness to carry on business as an optometrist, dispensing optician, or both. The GOC in order to fulfil this requirement issued in 2005 the Code of Conduct for Individual Registrants and the Code of Conduct for Business Registrants. Although not statutory documents these provided an outline of what the GOC expected from registrants. The Codes were reviewed on an annual basis and the Council agreed, as part of its 2008–9 and 2009–10 business plans, that a major review should be undertaken to ensure that the principles within them continued to be relevant, up to date, and reflect best regulatory practice.

The Standards Committee were tasked with overseeing the review and in April 2008 established a working group consisting of optometrist, dispensing optician, lay and business registrant members to undertake a detailed review of the Codes. In November 2008, on the recommendation of the Standards Committee, the Council approved for consultation a document outlining several proposals as to how the Codes might be amended. These documents were then put out for a three-month consultation period from January to April 2009. Following review of the consultation responses and further work by the Standards Committee the Codes of conduct for individual registrants and for business registrants were agreed by Council and published as standards in 2010.

These standards were in place for 5-years before the GOC considered that the existing Code of Conduct once more lacked detail and no longer met the needs of the profession. As a result, a standards strategic review and consultation exercise was undertaken, with three key objectives:

- To clarify, and ensure, that the statutory role of promoting high standards, including the role of providing guidance was fulfilled.
- To ensure that the standards of ethics and performance focus on outcomes, meet the public's expectations, are clear to registrants and reflect good practice.
- To ensure that the standards of competence and system of regulation in the interest of patient and public benefit enabled positive developments in optical practice.

Stakeholders were initially asked to consider how the scope of practise of optometrists and dispensing opticians may evolve in the future, and how standards should therefore adapt to ensure continuing patient safety. Research was carried out also into patient expectations. Additional consultation took place over 12 weeks (March–June 2015) and focused on the development of the standards framework and standards for optometrists, dispensing opticians, and optical students. The outcome of the consultation was publication by the GOC in 2016 of *Standards of Practice for Optometrists and Dispensing Opticians* and separate *Standards of*

Practice for Optical Students. New *Standards of Practice for Business Registrants* followed in Oct 2019.

Current Standards

The Standards of Practice for Optometrists and Dispensing Opticians define the standards of behaviour and performance expected of all registrants and are designed to make these expectations clear to professionals and patients. The GOC also consider that the standards give room for registrants to use their professional judgement in deciding how to apply them in any given situation.

There are 19 separate standards for registrants, but for students only 18 as continuing education is not considered relevant prior to qualification. The standards published by the GOC are not listed in order of priority and are presented in the form of a summary statement heading with additional more detailed clarification/expansion bullet points. The 19 standards headings for registered optometrists and dispensing opticians are listed in Table 1.

Table 1:   GOC Standards for registrants

- Listen to patients and ensure they are at the heart of the decisions made about their care
- Communicate effectively with your patients
- Obtain valid consent
- Show care and compassion for your patients
- Keep your knowledge and skills up to date
- Recognise, and work within, your limits of competence
- Conduct appropriate assessments, examinations, treatments, and referrals
- Maintain adequate patient records
- Ensure that supervision is undertaken appropriately and complies with the law
- Work collaboratively with colleagues in the interests of patients
- Protect and safeguard patients, colleagues, and others from harm
- Ensure a safe environment for your patients
- Show respect and fairness to others and do not discriminate
- Maintain confidentiality and respect your patients' privacy
- Maintain appropriate boundaries with others
- Be honest and trustworthy
- Do not damage the reputation of your profession through your conduct
- Respond to complaints effectively
- Be candid when things have gone wrong

In addition, the GOC published Standards for Optical Businesses that define the standards expected of optical businesses to protect the public and promote high standards of care. Although directed at businesses registered with the GOC the expectation is that the standard will apply to all providers in the optical sector. The standards are designed to map 3 areas covering patients, governance and staff and are shown below:

As a registered optical business you must ensure that, in relation to:

- *Your patients:*
  - o *Patients can expect to be safe in your care;*
  - o *Patient care is delivered in a suitable environment;*
  - o *Communication is clear and effective; and*
  - o *Patients can give valid consent to treatment.*
- *Your culture and governance:*
  - o *The services you provide are open and transparent;*
  - o *You ensure compliance with relevant regulations;*
  - o *You have a system of clinical governance in place; and*
  - o *Confidentiality is respected.*
- *Your staff:*
  - o *Staff are able to exercise their professional judgment;*
  - o *Staff are suitably trained, qualified and registered;*
  - o *Staff are adequately supervised; and*
  - o *Staff collaborate with others, where appropriate.*

College Guidance

The GOC remains the statutory body for optometric practice and therefore may take action against any registered optometrist where it feels that statutory requirements have not been met. The College of Optometrists, on the other hand, is a professional organization the aim of which is to maintain, for the public benefit, the highest possible standard of professional competence and conduct and as such it can take action only against its own members. There is a separate process for the College to consider breaches of their guidance by Fellows/members. Although the GOC will take note of the College of Optometrists guidance in any action taken against a practitioner both it and the Courts could override the College view if it were to be shown to differ from that of the reasonably competent "average" practitioner under similar circumstances or was not consistent with the GOC Standards of Practice.

The effect of withdrawal of the GOC N22 in 1987 at that time placed greater demands on the guidelines of The College of Optometrists and in order to meet the demands and fully to take the place of N22 a complete revision of the guidelines was undertaken resulting in the 1991 publication of the updated *The College Code of Ethics and Guidance for Professional Conduct.*

This set of guidelines was reviewed by other optical organisations such as the Federation of Ophthalmic and Dispensing Opticians, the Federation of Independent British Optometrists and the Association of Optometrists before publication and amended to take account of points raised where this was a general opinion. The result of this activity was guidance that took account of the views of all major optometric organisations and represented a consensus. The guidance has been reviewed subsequently at regular intervals and is seen by the College of Optometrists as an ongoing project.

Due to legislative changes and consumer attitudes the 1991 Guidelines rapidly became out of date and in 1997 the College of Optometrists released details of updated guidance specifically relating to the Routine Eye examination. The update however was in a different format to previous guidance and provided advice on BEST practice. While this was very laudable and provided a target to which every practitioner could aspire and self-assess it was not a peer view of current practice and created problems for the GOC when attempting to use them as a "peer view". The result was to create friction within the profession and the College agreed to review the guidelines. There have been many re-iterations of the guidance since then and the College has maintained a rolling review and involved representatives from other optometric organisations in developing its guidance over time. In 2014 the College removed the section on Ethics and produced an updated *Guidance for Professional Practice* in addition at this time *Clinical Management Guidelines* were published relating to diagnosis and management of a range of ocular conditions.

The latest version can be found on the College of Optometrists website at: http://www.college-optometrists.org.

In addition to clinical guidance the College provides an ethical Code of Conduct that all Fellows and Members sign up to. This has changed over time but currently provides 7 elements:

- Exercise your professional judgement and use your professional skills to the best of your ability.
- Discharge your professional responsibilities with integrity, considering and acting in the public interest when appropriate.
- Be an example of good practice to your colleagues.
- Do all in your power to ensure that your professional activities do not put the health and safety of others at risk.
- Never engage in any corrupt or unethical practice.
- Never engage in any activity that will impair the dignity and reputation of the College, fellow members, or the optometric profession.
- Observe the College's values when dealing with College employees, fellow members, your colleagues, and patients.

The guidance that the College issues represents its view of how the code of ethics should be interpreted by fellows and members in their professional lives and currently covers four main areas and includes 4 annexes. The main areas covered fall into:

- Knowledge, skills, and performance
- Safety and quality
- Communication, partnership, and teamwork
- Maintaining trust

The four Annexes cover:

- Annex 1 Equipment list for the routine eye examination
- Annex 2 Ophthalmic abbreviations
- Annex 3 World Health Organization guidance on hand rubbing and handwashing techniques
- Annex 4 Urgency of referrals table

What happens to Optometrists acting against the College guidelines?

These comprehensive sets of standards and guidelines are aimed at maintaining the high standard of patient care that is expected within the UK by all patients. The steps that may be taken by the GOC to investigate and discipline an optometrist for alleged offences have been outlined in Chapter 13. Ultimately, the GOC may erase a practitioner's name from the register and, therefore, prevent them from practising. The College has a more flexible approach to the problem, and although a formal investigation and disciplinary procedure can be undertaken, this is rarely required. The College can remove membership from an individual, but this does not prevent that individual from continuing to practice as an optometrist.

College Process for Dealing with a Complaint against a Fellow or Member

Complaints must be made in writing to the Chief Executive, and contain the full name of, and enough detail to verify the identity of, the Complainant and an account of the facts alleged against the Respondent which might constitute a breach of the Code of Conduct. The College may also raise a complaint about an individual via the Chief Executive or an Officer of the College. The Council of the College has delegated authority to the Chief Executive to decide whether a complaint requires investigation or not.

Where it is decided that a complaint should be followed-up the Chief Executive should notify the respondent in writing and request comments providing at least 28 days for a response. If it is decided that further investigation is then required, an investigating officer will be appointed, and a report prepared no later than 3 months after the appointment. At the conclusion of the investigation, the Chief Executive writes to the Respondent inviting him or her to comment within a set time on all the evidence gathered. Based on the evidence and any comments from the Respondent, the Chief Executive decides as to whether there is a realistic prospect that the Professional Conduct Committee will find the facts proven on the balance of probabilities and therefore that the member has breached the Code of Conduct.

If the Chief Executive decides either that there is not a realistic prospect of the facts being established by the Professional Conduct Committee, and/or that it is not in the best interests of the College to refer the complaint to the Professional Conduct Committee to determine, that will be the end of the investigation, and all parties informed accordingly.

Any decision by the Chief Executive not to refer to the Professional Conduct Committee is only taken with the agreement of the Chair of the Board of Trustees and Chair of the Professional Conduct Committee.

The Chief Executive may consider alternative courses of action including:

- issuing a warning to the Member, and when appropriate, providing support through either the College's Clinical Advice Service or directing the Member to relevant training and/or development;
- issuing a warning to the Member against any recurrence of the conduct which formed the basis of the complaint; or
- obtaining an appropriate undertaking from the Member.

Once a decision has been made to refer the matter to the Professional Conduct Committee the Chief Executive must make the necessary arrangements for the meeting to take place normally within three months of the decision to refer the complaint to the Professional Conduct Committee.

Once a meeting has been called the Respondent should be sent by special delivery or equivalent:

- notice of the date of the meeting
- a request to attend the meeting
- notification setting out the particulars of the complaint and a summary of evidence on which the complaint is based
- copies of any witness statements and documentary evidence provided to the Professional Conduct Committee
- a copy of the procedures.

The Respondent will be invited to submit a written statement, which in the absence of the Respondent at the meeting would be considered by the Professional Conduct Committee. Any such statement must be submitted at least 7 clear days prior to the meeting. In addition, the Respondent should be made aware that the Professional Conduct Committee may deal with the matter and impose a sanction in the Respondent's absence from the meeting.

Should the Committee decide that the complaint is upheld and there has been a Breach of College Guidance and after taking into account any mitigation submitted it decides in private on the sanction (if any) to be imposed on the Respondent. If the Respondent is present at the meeting and mitigation is presented the Professional Conduct Committee announces its decision orally if the Respondent is not present at the meeting, the Professional Conduct Committee considers any statement of mitigation as soon as reasonably practicable after it has been received and gives the Respondent written notice of its decision.

Potential Sanctions

The sanctions open to the committee are to:

- require the Respondent to undertake specified training and / or development appropriate to the breach in question in a form and within a time period as required by the Professional Conduct Committee, failing which some other sanction shall take effect, or the undertaking may be required as well as another sanction
- reprimand orally and in writing the Respondent
- suspend the Respondent from Membership of the College
- expel the Respondent from Membership of the College

When the Professional Conduct Committee has ordered the suspension or expulsion of a Member, the Member must immediately upon the sanction coming into effect, surrender his/her Certificate of Membership of the College, and for the period of his/her suspension or expulsion shall not be entitled to:

- state or give any indication that s/he is a Member
- use any affix to his/her name indicating possession of a qualification awarded by the College
- attend or vote at any General Meeting of the College
- serve on any committee of the College
- exercise or enjoy any other rights or privileges of a Member.

The Chief Executive notifies the Registrar of the GOC of the suspension or expulsion of any Member so that amendments can be made to the appropriate register.

GOC/College Fitness to Practise Procedures Pre 2005

The General Optical Council decided in 1997 that there were cases in which the Investigating Committee did not wish to refer the practitioner to the Disciplinary Committee but that there was concern about specific aspects of the practitioner's professional practise. To overcome this an informal and voluntary procedure for dealing with fitness to practice was introduced in conjunction with the College of optometrists. The role of the College was to provide support and advice for the practitioner to help to avoid similar problems in the future.

The College suggested the benefits of this fitness to practise procedure from the optometrist's perspective were:

- The practitioner had the opportunity to review his or her actions in discussion with peers, with the sole objective of highlighting problem areas and avoiding future difficulties
- The practitioner was given positive and constructive help, in a non-confrontational setting
- Where appropriate, practical training was arranged or courses recommended, to help enhance skills for future practice

It suggested from the GOC's perspective:

- The GOC could tackle matters of concern that were not necessarily appropriate for the statutory disciplinary process

- Public protection was safeguarded since perceived deficiencies in practice were addressed.

The process involved was simple and straightforward. After receiving details from the GOC, the College invited the practitioner concerned to attend the College to discuss the professional and clinical aspects of the case with the Professional Adviser and as it was at that time the Secretary. The advice and any recommendations resulting from the interview were ratified by the College's Professional Conduct Committee and confirmed in writing to the practitioner. The College monitored implementation of any recommended action and once a satisfactory outcome had been achieved a report was made to the GOC indicating a satisfactory conclusion.

The College website indicated that as of December 2000, 32 cases had been dealt with through this procedure. Some examples of the types of cases reviewed appeared in the optical press (Taylor & Edwards 1999).

This process however became redundant with the introduction of the new GOC Fitness to Practice procedure in 2005 — see Chapter 13.

Additional Advice from the GOC

In support of its standards for practice the GOC (and the professional bodies) has issued additional guidance on a series of topics.

Duty of Candour

The Health and Social Care Act 2008 (Regulated Activities) Regulations 2014 (SI 2014 2936) came into effect in November of that year and regulation 20 introduced statutory requirements for candour for NHS bodies as organisations, however it excluded primary care contractors and individual performers.

In October 2014 having had sight of the draft Bill the General Optical Council (GOC) joined seven other healthcare regulators in pledging in a joint statement to put openness and honesty at the heart of healthcare. This was to be achieved by including Candour requirements in their professional standards. The GOC also issued a statement saying:

"A 'duty of candour' for optometrists and dispensing opticians will mean they must be open and honest with patients when something goes wrong with their treatment or care which causes, or has the potential to cause, harm or distress."

The GOC as discussed above issued new Standards of Practice effective from April 2016 and these included a section dedicated to professional duty of candour (section19). The standard was consistent with the standards for candour published by the other 7 healthcare regulatory organisations. The standard applies to all registrants with the GOC including business registrants.

The result is that all healthcare professionals have a professional duty of candour that means they have a professional responsibility to be open, honest, and transparent with patients when things go wrong. The General Optical Council's *Standards of Practice for Optometrists and Dispensing Opticians* (standard 19) and *Standards for Optical Students* (standard 18) reflect this professional duty of candour.

The professional duty of candour applies when a healthcare professional becomes aware that something has gone wrong and as a result a patient in their care has suffered physical or psychological harm or distress, or their future care may be impacted as a result. For optometrists this could range from relatively minor incidents such as use of incorrect eyedrops to more serious issues such as failure to detect pathology.

Meeting the duty of candour means being open and honest and contacting the patient about what has gone wrong as soon as possible after an error has been picked-up. GOC guidance (Supplementary Guidance on the professional Duty of Candour) states:

"The patient must be told:
- *that something has gone wrong;*
- *what happened;*
- *the likely short and long term effects;*
- *what can be done to put matters right; and*
- *what can be done to avoid reoccurrence and improve patient care."*

An apology should be offered to express regret for any harm, distress or adverse consequences to the patient's health and wellbeing resulting from the incident. Saying sorry however does not mean admitting liability or wrongdoing. Offering an apology is an important part of being candid as it shows recognition of the impact of the situation on the patient and displays empathy.

When speaking to a patient the GOC guidance suggests the following should be considered:

"a. You must share information in a way that the patient can understand.
b. You should give information that the patient may find distressing in a considerate way, for example, asking them if they would like to have someone with them.
c. You should respect your patient's right to privacy and dignity, making sure that conversations take place in appropriate settings where possible.
d. If there is an on-going investigation you should be clear that the facts have not yet been established. Tell them only what you know and believe to be true and answer any questions honestly and as fully as you can.
e. You should make sure the patient knows whom to contact to ask any further questions or raise concerns.
f. You should record the details of your apology in the patient's clinical record. In certain circumstances, a verbal apology may need to be followed up by a written apology."

Sometimes an adverse event may occur that had the potential to cause harm or distress but was avoided and where no harm occurred and will not cause harm later. Professional judgement should be used when considering whether to inform patients about such events. In some situations, telling a patient of what might have occurred may distress or confuse them unnecessarily.

As with all adverse events consideration should be given as to why the event happened and what action should be taken in future to prevent reoccurrence by sharing learning to help ensure patient safety.

Consent

Section 3 of the GOC standards for practice relate to consent as shown below:

3.1 Obtain valid consent before examining a patient, providing treatment or involving patients in teaching and research activities. For consent to be valid it must be given:

3.1.1 Voluntarily.

3.1.2 By the patient or someone authorised to act on the patient's behalf.

3.1.3 By a person with the capacity to consent.

3.1.4 By an appropriately informed person. "Informed" means explaining what you are going to do and ensuring that patients are aware of any risks and options in terms of examination, treatment, sale and supply of optical appliances or research they are participating in. This includes the right of the patient to refuse treatment or have a chaperone or interpreter present.

3.2 Be aware of your legal obligations in relation to consent, including the differences in the provision of consent for children, young people and vulnerable adults. When working in a nation of the UK, other than where you normally practise, be aware of any differences in consent law and apply these to your practice.

3.3 Ensure that the patient's consent remains valid at each stage of the examination or treatment and during any research in which they are participating."

In support of the standard the GOC has issued additional guidance on consent. It is considered that patients have the right to determine what happens to their own bodies and make informed choices in healthcare and it is a general legal and ethical principle that valid consent must be obtained at the point of care and throughout treatment. Valid consent therefore is a fundamental part of good practice.

Consent takes various forms and patients can give consent in a variety of ways, all of which are considered as equally valid.

Explicit consent

This is when a patient gives specific permission for something to be done and can be either oral or written. Explicit consent should be obtained where the procedure, treatment or care being proposed requires for example physical contact with the patient and/or has greater risks involved.

Implied consent

This is when consent can be assumed from a patient's actions, for example, by placing their chin on an instrument's chin rest following an explanation of the test involved. Professional judgement must be used to decide what type of consent is required, taking into account the individual patient's needs, expressed expectations and circumstances, as well as the associated risks.

Voluntary consent

Voluntary consent applies to a decision to consent or not to consent made by the patient themselves based on informed consideration. Patients must not be coerced by healthcare professionals, relatives, or others to accept a particular type of treatment or care, or in the sale and supply of optical appliances. This is particularly important in situations in which patients may be vulnerable, for example, in domiciliary settings.

Informed consent

Obtaining consent is part of an on-going discussion and decision-making process between clinician and patient rather than something that happens in isolation. It is important therefore to be satisfied that the patient has in some way consented to all aspects of the care being providing. As part of the process of obtaining consent the patient should be provided with clear and accurate information in a way that they can understand. This may be in writing, including in a leaflet, or by talking to the patient, whether before or during their appointment.

Consent cannot be implied simply on the basis of a patient having attended an appointment, as the patient may not be sufficiently informed to provide valid consent. Consent also cannot be presumed because it was given on a previous occasion. A patient's consent must be obtained on each occasion that it is needed, for example, when there is a change in treatment or service options.

Valid consent

For consent to be valid it must be given by someone with the capacity to consent. 'Capacity' refers to a patient's ability to understand and retain information relevant to the decision required relating to their treatment or care, weigh up the information provided and the options available and communicate their decision.

Most adults are presumed to have the capacity to consent but there is a legal framework across the UK outlining how capacity is assessed in adults, young people, and children. When assessing capacity, the assessment should be objective and no assumption made that a patient lacks capacity based just upon their age, disability, beliefs, condition, or behaviour, or because they make a decision you disagree with.

Because a patient lacks capacity on one occasion, or in relation to one type of service, it should not be assumed that they lack capacity to make all decisions or the capacity to make decisions at all times. A patient's capacity to consent may be temporarily affected by a variety of other factors, for example, illness, prescribed medication, shock, panic, fatigue, confusion, pain or the effects of drugs or alcohol. In some circumstances therefore it may be appropriate to defer the decision on treatment until the temporary effects subside and capacity is restored.

If a patient is not able to make decisions for themselves the law sets out the criteria and processes to be followed and this may include the granting of legal authority to certain people to make decisions on behalf of patients who lack capacity.

In situations where a patient refuses or withdraws consent details of the reasons given by the patient for the decision and any discussions should be recorded on the patient notes.

Consent to share information

Information in a patient's record is subject to professional, ethical, and legal duties of confidentiality (See Chapter 12 for information on data protection). Most patients understand and expect that some confidential information will be shared between health and social care professionals as part of the care providing process.

According to the GOC guidance Optometrists may assume implied consent to share confidential information with those who are providing (or supporting the provision of) direct care to the patient when satisfied that all of the following apply:

a. the person accessing or receiving the information is providing or supporting the patient's care;
b. information is readily available to patients explaining how their information will be used (for example, in leaflets, posters, on websites or face to face), and they have the right to object;
c. the patient has not objected; and
d. that anyone to whom confidential information is disclosed understands that it is given to them in confidence, which they must respect.

Patients should not be surprised to learn about how their personal information is being used, accessed or disclosed and have the right for their wishes to be respected if they object to particular personal information being shared unless disclosure would be justified in the public interest, is required by law, or it is in the best interests of a patient who lacks capacity to make the decision in order to prevent harm.

Whistleblowing

The GOC have established a mechanism to raise public interest concerns, where it has not been possible to raise or resolve those concerns through internal processes. They cannot provide legal protection, but they can provide support and advice about raising concerns. Guidance has been produced covering raising concerns and making protected disclosures.

Protected disclosures can be made to the GOC on matters relating to:

- the registration of individuals and businesses registered with the GOC;
- the fitness to practise (FTP) of individuals and businesses registered with the GOC; and/or

- any other activities in relation to which the GOC have functions (including education and training, and illegal practice).

Issues related to personal grievances, disciplinary matters, contractual disputes, or other aspects of the working relationship, which should be managed informally or formally through the organisation's grievance policy are not covered in this process.

The GOC provide the following list of potential allegations of wrong-doing/malpractice at work which include, but are not limited to:

- criminal offences;
- failure to comply with an obligation set out in law;
- miscarriages of justice;
- endangering of someone's health and safety; and/or
- covering up wrongdoing in the above categories.

This can include individuals or organisations practising illegally, putting someone's health at risk through fitness to practise concerns, fraud, and financial impropriety.

Such concerns must be made in the public interest and the person raising the concern must reasonably believe that the information is substantially true.

The *Public Interest Disclosure Act 1998* (PIDA) gives legal protection to those raising concerns against detrimental treatment or dismissal as a result of disclosing information which is in the public interest. The Act offers a right to redress in the event of victimisation.

Chapter 16

The Negligent Professional

The law of tort covers many areas but the most common to impact on optometry practice is that of negligence. While many people will have their own concept of negligence, in law it has been clearly defined as:

> "A breach by the defendant of a legal duty of care which is owed to the plaintiff among others and breach of which causes damage to the plaintiff."

This mirrors the type of consideration the GOC or the NHS would give to a complaint from a patient i.e., it must be proven on "the balance of probabilities" and not "beyond reasonable doubt" see Chapter 13. "Beyond reasonable doubt" is the legal standard of proof required to find a defendant guilty in a British criminal trial and was required at one point in professional regulation. The major difference between professional regulation relating to negligence and civil law is that in a civil lawsuit if negligence is proven, damages will be awarded to the plaintiff.

Is negligence easy to demonstrate?

At face value the definition above seems clear enough and indeed to succeed in an action for negligence the plaintiff is required only to prove the following three conditions:

1. A duty of care is owed personally by the defendant to the plaintiff
2. The duty of care has been broken
3. Harm has been suffered as a result of the breach of duty

As always with the law, however, it is not quite so easy to prove the conditions.

Duty of care

To prove a duty of care is owed it is necessary to show that a defendant could reasonably have been expected to have foreseen that a person such as the plaintiff might have been affected by his act or failure to act. The duty of care however can take several forms:

Contractual duty of care

In this situation there should be clear evidence of the duty of care owed. If for example an optometrist is registered as a provider with NHS England to provide GOS sight testing on its behalf, then when undertaking such tests, a clear duty of care has been established. If, however an optometrist is contracted by an employer to test for example only the pressure of all the employees and identify any with raised intraocular pressure failure to detect a cataract would not necessarily constitute a breach of duty of care as it did not form part of the contract and may not have been obvious through the test being performed.

General duty of care

In the case of optometry or dispensing optics if a qualified practitioner sees a patient in practice, that patient would expect the practitioner to carry out their duties with care beyond that expected from an ordinary reasonable person. If a practitioner sets up as a 'specialist' in a particular field such as contact lenses any patient would expect the practitioner to carry out any duties with care beyond that expected from an 'ordinary' optometrist. It is well established in law that a duty of care does exist between the practitioner and patient even though there may be no specific contract or agreement.

The general duty of care however could extend beyond the individual patient seen. For example, a practitioner uses eye drops that reduce a patient's vision but does not warn the patient of the risks of driving until vision is back to normal. On leaving the practice the patient drives away and is involved in a traffic accident with a third party — the duty of care owed by the practitioner could be seen to extend to the third party.

The logic behind this interpretation is that the practitioner should know that the patient with reduced vision could be dangerous when driving and could therefore foresee the potential for an accident. If however the practitioner gives adequate warning to the patient and the patient ignores the advice given the practitioner could be seen to have completed his duty of care.

Several attempts have been made to define the principle of duty of care and the definition normally quoted is that given by Lord Atkins in Donoghue v Stevenson in 1932. It is sometimes called the "Neighbour principle" and simply says that a duty of care exists when parties are involved in a close and proximate relationship, where one party can reasonably foresee that by his action, he is likely to cause harm to the other party.

Breach of duty

Once it has been established that a duty of care existed between the practitioner and the plaintiff it still has to be proved that the duty of care was broken, and that the behaviour of the defendant was sufficiently careless as to make it reasonably foreseeable that some injury to the plaintiff might result.

The courts will expect qualified practitioners to exercise skill and care above that which the courts would expect of an ordinary reasonable person. In assessing whether a practitioner's conduct has fallen below the expected standard the court will look to the opinion of those practitioners of a similar standing. If the practitioner professes a specialist skill (e.g., contact lenses) the standard expected would be higher than for a non-specialist but qualified practitioner.

This is the area where the court in order to determine expectation could use the standards of practice issued by the GOC and guidelines issued by the College of Optometrists. The court must be satisfied that the practitioner behaves as would an average practitioner of similar standing and it becomes important to distinguish between "best" practice and "normal" practice. It would be for the court to listen to arguments and then decide on whether the College guidelines represented an average view and are representative of what a patient might realistically expect.

The issue of experience is also relevant here. It has been determined that should a newly qualified practitioner undertake a particular procedure that practitioner will be judged on the same standards as an experienced practitioner performing the same procedure — no allowance is made for lack of training. In this way the duty is "tailored to the act not the actor". As practitioners are expected to work within the limitations of their abilities the newly qualified would be required to demonstrate the skills etc that would be required to perform the particular task.

A court will not automatically consider a practitioner liable if a diagnosis is incorrect. What is expected is that due care and skill has gone into arriving at the decision. It is therefore important to understand when further diagnostic tests are necessary and when referral to a specialist is the most suitable option. It is also important to carefully record all activity.

Harm has been suffered

As mentioned above duty of care, breach of duty and harm arising must be proven for action on negligence to succeed. It doesn't matter how careless a course of action may be if no harm results there is no liability.

The breach of duty may not need to be the sole contributory factor to the harm resulting but must have materially contributed. The general rule for the standard of proof in all civil cases is "but for the defendant's fault, on the balance of probabilities, the injury complained of would not have occurred". In essence this means the plaintiff must persuade the court that there was a greater than 50% chance that the action of the defendant resulted in harm.

Let us look at the example of a patient attending for examination with a small retinal detachment. A cursory examination is carried out and the detachment is not noted. The following day the detachment increases, and the patient attends a casualty unit and is treated so that no permanent damage results. In this case it is likely that detecting the detachment one day earlier would have made little difference to the outcome and negligence may be hard to prove. If, however, the patient assumes that all is well after the visit to the optometrist and does not attend the casualty but continues for two weeks before seeking a further opinion it could be very different. The detachment is enlarged and reaching the macula area and re attachment now becomes difficult resulting in permanent damage to the retina. In this case the original practitioner could be considered liable for negligence.

In 2016 for the first time an optometrist was found guilty of the criminal charge of gross negligence manslaughter — this was based on an instance of missed pathology where a patient subsequently died. The verdict was overturned on appeal, but it demonstrates the potential extent to which legal action may cover.

Damages

"Damages" is the financial measure of the harm suffered. When considering a case, the court will attempt to ensure that the injured party is maintained in the position that they would have been had the harm not occurred. Normally consideration will be given to two aspects the first relating to matters leading up to the case reaching court e.g., loss of earnings, special equipment purchases, medical expenses etc. and the second dealing with future financial loss. The first is relatively easy to determine the second is not.

When considering the future, the court will try to put a figure to:

- Compensation for pain and suffering resulting from the harm
- Effect on enjoyment of life
- Future loss of earnings
- Loss of earnings capacity and prospects
- Loss of benefits such as pension
- Future expenses including medical care

Period of action

It can often take some time before the results of a particular action or failed action become apparent and, while mindful of this, the Law is also aware of the strain of waiting. To provide an equitable solution, the law provides a time frame within which action may be taken. There is a limit of three years starting either from the date on which the action occurred or the date on which harm as a result of the action became apparent. It is possible for a court to allow action beyond this period, but the circumstances would need to be exceptional.

In the case of a minor there is a further variation, and the 3-year period commences from their eighteenth birthday when they attain majority.

Protection from Claims

It is not possible to achieve complete protection from the possibility of a claim for negligence being brought against a practitioner. To minimise the risk a practitioner can either

1. Carry out every test on every patient and ensure that all the minor variations in results are accountable
2. Refer every patient with even the most minor of problems
3. Complete a thorough routine using tests to investigate symptoms and observations of the patient and to support results found and recorded during an examination.

The first two options are not sustainable in a real practice situation leaving the third one as the only realistic mode of practice. A practitioner taking the Russian roulette view that "it will never happen to me" is not minimising risk in any way and is open to action at any time.

It is for this reason that insurance is necessary to cover the risk of a claim occurring. In some case the amounts awarded in damages can run to seven figures enough to affect most optometrists if they had to raise the funds themselves! The issue of indemnity insurance will be addressed in Chapter 17.

Chapter 17

The Need for Insurance

The implications of civil action were discussed in Chapter 16 with particular reference to negligence claims. To protect yourself as an optometrist and to ensure financial support for any damages due to a patient succeeding in an action it is normal to take out some form of indemnity insurance. Insurance cannot alter the decision of a court or a professional body, but it can provide the finances to fight a case where insurers deem it appropriate and provide a sum to cover the cost of damages awarded where appropriate.

As the frequency of litigation increases and the value of damages awarded increases, so the cost of insurance is likely to increase. Competition is fierce however within the insurance industry and often as premiums rise the range of benefits offered is also improved.

Who needs professional insurance?

Any qualified member of the profession should have a form of professional liability insurance and it is a requirement for registration with the GOC. The Health Act 1999 provided the Secretary of State for Health with an enabling power to introduce a law requiring all professionals to have liability cover. If you are in practice and therefore come into contact with members of the public, you are at risk of making an error during your career and potentially action being taken for negligence. As set out in Chapter 16 even the most careful of practitioners can err or misjudge.

In 2005 it became a requirement of annual registration with the GOC that adequate insurance is in place, and this is incorporated into the Standards of Practise section 12.2 which states that a registrant must:

"Have adequate professional indemnity insurance and only work in practices that have adequate public liability insurance. This includes the following:

12.2.1 If insurance is provided by your employer, you must confirm that adequate insurance is in place.

12.2.2 If you work in multiple practices, you must ensure that there is adequate insurance to cover each working environment.

12.2.3 Your professional indemnity insurance must provide continuous cover for the period you are in practise."

12.2.4 Your professional indemnity insurance must cover complaints that are received after you stop practising, as these might be received years later — this is sometimes referred to as 'run-off' cover."

What type of insurance should I have?

in the case of professional liability, it is sensible to take out insurance covering four main aspects:

1. Professional liability cover:
   This is legal liability cover in respect of advice given for a fee. It should be noted however that if you act as an expert witness you may need to increase the level of and/or modify the terms of your policy to ensure adequate cover.
2. Products liability cover
   This is legal liability that can arise from accidental injuries sustained by or accidental loss of or damage to the property of a third party arising from defects in goods sold or supplied or from the repair, servicing, cleaning, or alteration of goods. An example of a claim made under this aspect would be for injury caused following a screw falling out of spectacles. The vast majority of patients survive such episodes intact but there is a risk of damage here.

3. Third party liability cover

    This may be defined as legal liability arising out of premises risks only. A claim made by a patient who had walked into an unsigned glass door within a practice and been injured would be an example of this type of claim.

4. Public liability including medical malpractice

    This cover relates to legal liability for third party bodily injury or disease and is by far the most common type of insurance claim made by optometrists. Examples of claims falling within this category range from missed pathology to damage following the provision of incorrect contact lens solutions.

It is essential to ensure that your policy includes cover for legal defence costs. Most policies of this nature would include the costs involved in defending an action brought by an individual patient. The insurance should also cover costs involved in dealing with a potential GOC or NHS case.

As the optometry profession develops over time it is important to be sure that your insurance cover adapts with the changes. If you are involved in special activities such as contracted care schemes it is worth talking to your insurance adviser about the need/costs of additional cover for these specialised situations that may fall outside the scope of normal optometric cover. While standard malpractice insurance should cover you for most eventualities that would crop up in a normal practice situation some activities (e.g., the use of therapeutics) may not be automatically included in a "standard" medical malpractice policy.

Where you act as an expert witness or provide specialist advice as mentioned earlier it may be that your standard professional liability insurance cover will need to be upgraded. In addition to an ophthalmic malpractice cover it may be necessary to take out a separate professional indemnity insurance. Frequently companies have blanket cover for situations that occur in a practice that would provide cover for an individual — this may however not be the most suitable type of insurance for all situations, and it is important particularly where services are supplied on a locum basis to clarify the position and to consider individual cover.

What happens if I stop work?

It is possible to take out two forms of professional liability insurance. The first is based on "occurrence" such that the insurer "on risk" at the time of the incident deals with the claim irrespective of when the claim is made. The second is based on "claims made" under which a claim is dealt with by the insurer that is "on risk" at the time the claim is made. The advantage of the "occurrence" format is that you are covered even after you decide to stop practising. In the case of "claims made" policies you would need to take out "run off" cover for claims that may occur after you have given up practise.

There is a further complication when you switch from "claims made" to "occurrence" format. You would be well advised to take out "retrospective cover" for the years leading up to the change. Most insurance advisers will be pleased to discuss these issues with you, and it is essential that you are clear in your own mind exactly which form of insurance you have.

How much cover should I take out?

This is obviously up to the individual and will vary over time but currently (2021) as an example Federation of Ophthalmic and Dispensing Opticians cover for medical malpractice is for 10 million pounds per event with a maximum annual amount and this is consistent with the level offered by the AOP.

When an individual is injured, and liability for the accident is found to lie with another party, the subsequent court case determines the amount of money in damages they receive to compensate for their loss. This loss relates to earnings and expenses and can extend to cover the rest of their life. Considered are age, life expectancy and the level of earnings received currently.

Often Insurance Companies will attempt to come to an agreement without the case going to court and this saves on potentially significant expenses and time. For many practitioners who consider themselves to be at no fault this can be extremely disconcerting. The fact that a case is settled by agreement without admission of liability is however a way of reducing potential costs and reducing the time scale over which the particular case may spread. This should reduce the inevitable pressure that builds on all those involved. This course of action may be taken when a successful defence action is considered uncertain for example due to poor record keeping.

Previous claims settled range from sums of a few hundred pounds covering costs and professional fees for solicitors to hundreds of thousands of pounds to provide an out of court settlement including compensation. As patients become more aware of their rights and the role of the practitioner as a detector of pathology and manager of conditions develops the number of claims could potentially increase and the level of settlement will certainly increase in line with inflation, care costs etc.

How great a risk is there?

The simple answer to this is too great a risk not to take out insurance cover hence the GOC requirement as a prerequisite for registration. The number of cases each year may be small in terms of the total number of patients seen but if you are the practitioner involved it can be devastating. The practitioner has to contend with the worry, the fall in confidence, the potential knock-on effect of bad publicity with other patients and the effect on family members. More than this there is also the time taken to finalise the case (sometimes it can take years before a resolution is agreed) and the time taken out of work to attend meetings and prepare information.

It is unlikely that the total number of claims to insurers made by the optical profession is accurately known. However, it has been estimated that less than 1 in 50000 eye examinations results in an insurance claim each year. Based on the average number of registrants over the last few years that means approximately 3 cases for each practitioner during their lifetime! This low number is not so surprising as minor disagreements and complaints will be sorted within the practice and only more serious cases will reach the insurer.

Many of the claims reaching insurers relate to failure to detect pathology or failure to take appropriate action when detected. Within this group in the past retinal detachment, cataract and glaucoma have been the most frequent pathologies identified. The two other major issues resulting in claims relate to contact lenses/incorrect contact lens solutions and incorrect prescriptions.

How do I get insured?

The professional organisations FODO, AOP and ABDO all offer insurance and where an individual is employed or working for a corporate body blanket insurance is available. If employed within the NHS there is a litigation insurance in place to cover most aspects of clinical care, but it is still advisable to review whether additional personal cover is needed.

If you do not wish to be part of these schemes, there are underwriting insurance companies that regularly advertise in the professional journals who will tailor insurance to your particular needs. Whoever provides your insurance should supply you with a detailed schedule of the cover provided and any exclusions — check this very carefully and make sure it meets your specific needs.

Remember that insurance cover is only provided for risk notified to the insurer and if you practise techniques which are not considered "normal" practise, or you provide services from premises not notified to the insurer you may invalidate any claim. The insurer is there to help, and any queries will normally be dealt with professionally and effectively.

The GOC requires registrants to confirm evidence of suitable insurance for initial registration and annual retention. The College of Optometry insists on a signed statement indicating that adequate insurance provision has been arranged as a requirement for continued membership. As stressed above if you are unsure of your position check with your employer or with your insurance provider — it is not worth the risk of being uninsured or underinsured.

Appendix

Optical Bodies and Associations

Association of British Dispensing Opticians

Represents qualified dispensing opticians. A regular magazine *Dispensing Optics* is published.

Unit 2 Court Lodge Offices
Godmersham Park
Godmersham
Kent CT4 7DT
www.abdo.org.uk

Association of Contact Lens Manufacturers

Representing the major manufacturers of contact lenses in the UK.

Simon Rodwell
PO Box 737
Devizes
Wilts SN10 3TQ
www.aclm.org.uk

Association of Optometrists (AOP)

Represents the political interests of the optometrist. Approximately half of all qualified optometrists are members. A regular magazine *Optometry Today* is published.

2 Woodbridge Street
London
EC1R 0DG
Tel: 02075492000
www.aop.org.uk

British Contact Lens Association

Ophthalmic opticians/optometrists and dispensing opticians with a special interest in contact lenses may join this association. A regular journal is published.

199 Gloucester Terrace
London
W2 6LD
Tel: 02075806661
www.bcla.org.uk

College of Optometrists

Representing over 90 per cent of qualified optometrists, the College maintains professional standards, organises professional examinations and monitors the academic standards of the profession. An International research journal, *Ophthalmic and Physiological Optics,* is published four times a year in addition to *Optometry in Practice* a continuing education journal and *Acuity* a regular member Journal.

42 Craven Street
LONDON
WC2 5NG
Tel: 0207 839 6000
www.college-optometrists.org

Department of Health

39 Victoria Street
London
SW1H 0EU
Tel: 020 7210 4850
www.gov.uk

Federation of Ophthalmic and Dispensing Opticians

FODO is a national association of eye care providers working in primary
and community care settings. Each year its members provide over 18 million eye examinations and offer a wide range of other eye care services
across the UK.

16 Upper Woburn Place
London
WC1H 0BS
Tel: 020 7298 5151
www.fodo.com

Royal College of Ophthalmologists

Representing consultants in Ophthalmology and those studying for
specialist qualifications in ophthalmology.

18 Stephenson Way
London
NW1 2HD
Tel: 02079350702

General Optical Council (GOC)

Established under the terms of the Opticians Act 1958, the GOC has a
duty to protect the public interest by setting required standards for the
ophthalmic optical/optometric profession.

10 Old Bailey
London
EC4M 7NG
Tel: 02075803898
www.optical.org

Health Service Ombudsman

Set up by Parliament to provide an independent complaint handling service for complaints that have not been resolved by the NHS in England. Powers are set out in the Health Service Commissioners Act 1993. The Ombudsman Service is not part of government or the NHS in England and neither a regulator nor a consumer champion.

London
Millbank Tower
21 Millbank
Westminster
London
SW1P 4QP

Manchester
Citygate
Mosley Street
Manchester
M2 3HQ
Tel Helpline: 03450154033

Institute of Optometry

A registered charity providing eyecare services, clinical research, and postgraduate training

56-62 Newington Causeway
London
SE1 6DS

Tel: 02072349641
www.ioo.org.uk

Optometry Northern Ireland

65 Sandown Road
Belfast
BT5 6GU
Tel: 02895363239
www.optometryni.co.uk

Optometry Scotland

Representative body of optometrists in Scotland representing the view of the optical sector in Scotland to the Scottish Parliament, the Scottish Government Health Directorates, and other relevant stakeholders.

Baltic Chambers
50 Wellington Street
Glasgow
G2 6HJ
Tel: 01412020611
www.optometryscotland.org.uk

Optometry Wales

Optometry Wales is the professional umbrella organisation for the primary care eye health profession in Wales. It represents and works on behalf of all community optometrists, opticians, and dispensing opticians across Wales.

21 Alexon Way
Alexander Place
Hawthorn
Nr Pontypridd

CF37 5BS
Tel: 01443400796
www.optometrywales.org.uk

Worshipful Company of Spectacle Makers (SMC)

The oldest established of the remaining professional organisations, this company now has forsaken its examining role in optometry and has become more involved with training in the optical manufacturing industry.

Apothecaries Hall
Blackfriars Lane
LONDON
EC4V 6EL
Tel: 020 7236 2932
www.spectaclemakers.com

Useful Regulation References

Statutes

National Health Service, Act 1946
National Health Service (Scotland) Act 1947
Health Services (Northern Ireland) Act 1947
Nurseries and Child-Minders Regulation Act 1948
National Assistance Act 1948
Companies Act 1948
National Health Service (Amendment) Act 1949
Shops Act 1950
National Health Service Act 1951
National Health Service Act 1952
Opticians Act 1958
Factories Act 1961
National Health Service Act 1961
Offices, Shops and Railway Premises Act 1963

Shops (Early Closing Days) Act 1965
Companies Act 1967
Misrepresentation Act 1967
Trade Descriptions Act 1968
Health Services and Public Health Act 1968
Medicines Act 1968
Employers Liability (Compulsory Insurance) Act 1969
Equal Pay Act 1970
Misuse of Drugs Act 1971
Fire Precautions Act 1971
Road Traffic Act 1972
National Health Service Reorganisation Act 1973
Health and Safety at Work etc. Act 1974.
Sex Discrimination Act 1975
National Health Service Act 1977
Criminal Law Act 1977
National Health Service (Scotland) Act 1978
Employment Protection (Consolidation) Act 1978
Sale of Goods Act 1979
Health Service Act 1980
Supreme Court Act 1981
Supply of Goods and Services Act 1982
Health and Social Security Act 1984
Data Protection Act 1984
Companies Consolidation (Consequential Provisions) Act 1985
National Health Service (Amendment) Act 1986
Health and Medicines Act 1988
Opticians Act 1989
National Health Service and Community Care Act 1990
Access to Health Records Act 1990
Social Security Administration Act 1992
Health Service Commissioners Act 1993
Sale and Supply of Goods Act 1994
Health Authorities Act 1995
Disability Discrimination Act 1995
Employment Rights Act 1996

The National Health Service (Primary Care) Act 1997
Data Protection Act 1998
The Public Interest Disclosure Act 1998
Health Act 1999
Freedom of Information Act 2000
Freedom of Information (Scotland) Act 2002
Health and Social Care Act 2001
NHS Reform and Health Care Professions Act 2002
NHS Act 2006
NHS Consequential Provisions Act 2006
Health Act 2006
Health and Social Care Act 2008
Health Act 2009
Health and Social Care Act 2012
Health and Social Care (Safety and Quality) Act 2015
Data Protection Act 2018

Statutory instruments

1922/731	Chemical Works Regulations
1953/1464	Iron and Steel Foundries Regulations
1956/1077	National Health Service (Service Committees and Tribunal) Regulations
1956/1078	National Health Service (Supplementary Ophthalmic Services) Regulations
1960/1932	Shipbuilding and Ship-Repairing Regulations
1960/1934	General Optical Council (Disciplinary Committee Roles) Order of Council
1960/1935	General Optical Council (investigating Committee Rules) Order of Council
1960/1936	General Optical Council (Rules Relating to Injury or Disease of the Eye) Order of Council
1961/1239	General Optical Council Disciplinary Committee (Legal Assessor) Rules
1961/1580	Construction (General Provisions) Regulations

1961/1933	General Optical Council (Disciplinary Committee) Procedure Order of Council
1962/1667	Non-ferrous metals (Melting and Founding Regulations)
1964/167	General Optical Council (Rules on Publicity) Order of Council
1965/1366	National Health Service (Service Committees and Tribunal) Amendment Regulations
1969/354	National Health Service (Service Committees and Tribunal) (Amendment) Regulations
1969/1826	General Optical Council (Disciplinary Committee) (Procedure) Order of Council
1974/287	National Health Service (General Ophthalmic Services) Regulations
1974/455	National Health Service (Service Committees and Tribunal) Regulations
1974/527	National Health Service (General Ophthalmic Services) (Amendment) Regulations
1974/907	National Health Service (Service Committees and Tribunal) Amendment Regulations
1974/1681	Protection of Eyes Regulations
1975/789	National Health Service (General Ophthalmic Services) (S.) (Amendment) Regulations
1976/303	Protection of Eyes (Amendment) Regulations
1976/968	The Medicines (Specified Articles and Substances) Order
1976/2010	Fire Precautions (Non-Certificated Factory, Office, Shop and Railway Premises) Regulations
1977/434	National Health Service (Charges and Remission) Amendment Regulations
1977/1999	National Health Service (General Ophthalmic Services) Amendment Regulations
1977/2127	Medicines (Prescription Only) Order
1977/2129	Medicines (General Sale List) Order
1977/2132	Medicines (Sale or Supply) (Miscellaneous Provisions) Regulations
1977/2133	Medicines (Pharmacy and General Sale — Exemption) Order

1978/950	National Health Service (Dental and Optical Charges) Regulations
1978/987	Medicines (Prescription Only) Amendment (No. 2) Order
1978/988	Medicines (Pharmacy and General Sale — Exemption) Amendment Order
1978/989	Medicines (Sale or Supply) (Miscellaneous Provisions) Amendment Regulations
1979/1114	Medicines (Exemption from Licences) (Assembly) Order
1979/1539	Medicines (Contact Lens Fluids and Other Substances) (Appointed Day) Order
1979/1585	Medicines (Contact Lens Fluids and Other Substances) (Exemption from Licences) Order
1980/1921	Medicines (Prescription Only) Order
1980/1922	Medicines (General Sale List) Order
1980/1923	Medicines (Sale or Supply) Miscellaneous Provisions Regulations
1980/1924	Medicines (Pharmacy and General Sale — Exemption) Order
1981/552	General Optical Council (Rules and Publicity) Order
1981/952	Motor Vehicle (Driving Licences) Regulations
1982/28	Medicines (Sale or Supply) (Miscellaneous Provisions) Amendment Regulations
1983/1212	Medicines (Products other than Veterinary Drugs) (Prescription Only) Order
1984/769	Medicines (Products other than Veterinary Drugs) (General Sales List) Order
1984/1778	Sale of Optical Appliances Order
1985/203	General Optical Council (Rules on Publicity) Order
19851298	National Health Service (General Ophthalmic Services) Amendment Regulations
1985/856	General Optical Council (Rules on the Fitting of Contact Lenses) Order
1985/2024	General Optical Council (Registration and Enrolment) (Amendment) (Rules) Order
1986/309	General Optical Council (Membership) Order

1986/974	Health and Social Security Act 1984 (Commencement No. 2) Order
1986/975	National Health Service (General Ophthalmic Service) Regulations
1986/976	National Health Service (Payments for Optical Appliances) Regulations
1986/1136	National Health Service (Payments for Optical Appliances Amendment Regulations
1988/428	National Health Service (Payments for Optical Appliances) Regulations
1988/486	National Health Service (General Ophthalmic Services) Amendment Regulations
1988/552	National Health Service (Payments for Optical Appliances) Amendment No. 2 Regulations
1988/1305	General Optical Council (Contact Lens (Qualifications, etc.) (Rules)) Order.
1989/375	General Optical Council (Contact Lens (Qualifications, etc.) ((Amendment) Rules)) Order of Council
1989/395	National Health Service (General Ophthalmic Services) Amendment Regulations
1989/791	The Contact Lens Specification Rules
1989/1230	Sight Testing (Examination and Prescription) (No. 2) Regulations
1989/1174	The Health and Medicines Act 1988 (Commencement No 5) Order
1989/1175	National Health Service (General Ophthalmic Services) Amendment No. 2 Regulations
1989/1176	Sight Testing (Examination and Prescription) Regulations General Optical Council (Specification) Rules Order of Council
1989/1852	Medicines (Prescription Only, Pharmacy and General Sale) Amendment Order
1990/495	National Health Service (Optical Charges and Payments) Amendment Regulations
1990/538	National Health Service (Service Committees and Tribunal) Amendment Regulations

1990/1051   The National Health Service (General Ophthalmic Services) Amendment Regulations

1990/1752   National Health Service, (Service Committees and Tribunal) Amendment (No. 2) Regulations

1991/824   European Communities (Recognition of Professional Qualifications) Regulations

1992/664   National Health Service (Service Committees and Tribunal) Regulations

1993/483   General Optical Council (Registration and Enrolment (Amendment) Rules)

1994/70   General Optical Council (Testing of Sight by Persons Training as Ophthalmic Opticians Rules)

1994/2579   General Optical Council (Companies Committee Rules) Order of Council

1995/558   National Health Service (General Ophthalmic Services) Amendment Regulations

1995/3091   National Health Service (Service Committees and Tribunal) Amendment Regulations

1996/703   National Health Service (Service committees and Tribunal) Amendment Regulations

1996/705   National Health Service (General Ophthalmic Services) Amendment Regulations

1996/2320   National Health Service (General Ophthalmic Services) Amendment (No") Regulations

1996/2374   European Communities (Recognition of Professional Qualifications) (Second General System) Regulations

1997/818   National Health Service (Optical Charges and Payments) Regulations

1997/1780   National Health Service (Primary Care) Act 1997 (Commencement No1) Order

1997/1830   Prescription only Medicines (Human Use) Order

1998/1337   General Optical Council (Disciplinary Committee (Procedure) (Amendment) Rules)

1998/1338   General Optical Council (Disciplinary Committee (Constitution) Rules)

1998/3117   General Optical Council (Membership)

2005/848	The Opticians Act 1989 (Amendment) Order 2005
2005/1473	The GOC (Continuing Education and Training) Rules
2005/1474	The General Optical Council (Committee Constitution Rules) Order of Council
2005/1475	The General Optical Council (Fitness to Practise Rules) Order of Council
2005/1476	The General Optical Council (Injury or Disease of the Eye and Contact Lens (Qualifications)) (Amendment) Rules Order of Council
2005/1477	The General Optical Council (Registration Appeals Rules) Order of Council
2005/1478	General Optical Council (Registration Rules) Order of Council
2005/1507	The Medicines for Human Use (Prescribing) (Miscellaneous Amendments) Order
2005/1520	The Medicines (Sale or Supply) (Miscellaneous Amendments) Regulations 2005 (SI 2005 No. 1520
2005/3324	The Medicines for Human Use (Prescribing) (Miscellaneous Amendments) (No 2) Order
2006/135	The National Health Service (General Ophthalmic Services) (Scotland) Regulations
2006/2901	The General Optical Council (Continuing Education and Training) (Amendment No2) Rules Order of Council
2007/2781	The European Communities (Recognition of Professional Qualifications) Regulations
2007/3101	The European Qualifications (Health and Social Care Professions Regulations
2007/3491	The National Health Service (Primary Medical Services) (Miscellaneous Amendments) Regulations 2007
2008/1161	The Medicines for Human Use (Prescribing) (Miscellaneous Amendments) Order 2008
2008/1162	The Medicines (Sale or Supply) (Miscellaneous Amendments) Regulations 2008
2008/1185	National Health Service, England General Ophthalmic Services Contracts Regulations
2008/1186	Primary Ophthalmic Services Regulations

2008/1187   The National Health Service (Performers Lists) Amendment and Transitional Provisions Regulations 2008

2008/1657   The NHS (Optical Charges and Payments) Amendment (No2) Regulations

2008/1940   The General Optical Council (Therapeutics and Contact Lens Specialities) Rules Order of Council

2008/2690   The General Optical Council (Fitness to Practise) (Amendment in Relation to Standard of Proof) Rules Order of Council

2008/3113   The General Optical Council (Committee Constitution) (Amendment) Rules Order of Council

2009/309   The Local Authority Social Services and National Health Service Complaints (England) Regulations

2009/442   Health Care and Associated Professions (Opticians) The General Optical Council (Constitution) Order

2010/76   The NHS (Functions of the First-tier Tribunal relating to Primary Medical, Dental and Ophthalmic Services) Regulations

2010/412   The National Health Service (Performers Lists) Amendment Regulations 2010

2010/2841   The Medical Profession (Responsible Officer) Regulations

2012/1916   The Human Medicines Regulations 2012

2012/2882   The General Optical Council (Continuing Education and Training Rules) (Amendment) Order of Council

2013/335   National Health Service (Performers Lists (PL)) (England) Regulations

2013/365   The National Health Service (Primary Ophthalmic Services) (Miscellaneous Amendments and Transitional Provisions) Regulations 2013

2013/461   National Health Service (Optical Charges and Payments) Regulations

2013/2537   The General Optical Council (Fitness to Practise) Rules Order of Council

2014/418   National Health Service (Primary Ophthalmic Services and Optical Payments) (Miscellaneous Amendments) Regulations

2014/2936	The Health and Social Care Act 2008 (Regulated Activities) Regulations
2015/238	The National Health Service (Charges to Overseas Visitors) Regulations 2015
2015/362	The National Health Service (Performers Lists) (England) (Amendment) Regulations 2015
2015/2059	European Union (Recognition of Professional Qualifications) Regulations 2015
2016/1030	The European Qualifications (Health and Social Care Professions) Regulations
2017/1056	National Health Service (Primary Dental Services and General Ophthalmic Services) (Amendment) Regulations European Union (General Data Protection requirements (Council Decision (EU) 2018/893))
2019/419	The Data Protection, Privacy and Electronic Communications (Amendments etc) (EU Exit) Regulations
2019/593	The European Qualifications (Health and Social Care Professions) (Amendment etc.) (EU Exit) Regulations
2020/1394	The European Qualifications (Health and Social Care Professions) (EFTA States) (Amendment etc.) (EU Exit) Regulations 2020

Book and Journal References

ANGEL, S & TAYLOR, S P (1999) Professional Insurance Cover. *Optician 218,* 5690 20–22

BELL, J (2000) Valid Clinical Reasons for Patient Re-examination — *Optometry Today* July 14, 2000, p 28–29

BOSLEY, S and DALE J, (2008) Healthcare assistants in general practice: Practical and conceptual issues of skill-mix change *Br J Gen Pract.* February 1; 58(547): 118–124.

CLASSE, J. G. (1989) Legal Aspects of Optometry (U.S.A), Butterworths, Boston

CURRAN, R (2017) Community Eyecare Services in Northern Ireland: putting the patient at the centre, improving outcomes and maximising system resource Eyenews UK Vol 24 issue 2 https://www.eyenews.uk.com/features/optometry/post/community-eyecare-services-in-northern-ireland-putting-the-patient-at-the-centre-improving-outcomes-and-maximising-system-resource

DOUGHTY, M. J. (1999) Drugs, Medications and the Eye. Butterworth Heinemann

GILES, G. H. (1953) The Ophthalmic Services under the National Health Service Acts 1946–1952, Hammonds, London

HIRJI, N. K. & CLARKSON, R (2006) The Opticians Act 1989 (Amendment) Order 2005 — So what is the story? *Contact Lens & Anterior Eye* 29, 217–220

HOPKINS, G & PEARSON, R (1998) Ophthalmic Drugs. Butterworth Heinemann

KOCH, C (1947) British Reaction to the National Health Insurance Scheme. *American Journal of Optometrists and Archives of the Academy of Optometrists*, 24, 151–169

McKENNA, H.P, HASSON, F, KEENEY, S (2004) Patient safety and quality of care: the role of the health care assistant. *J Nurs Manag* 12(6):452–9.

MOJA L & KWAG KH (2015) Point of care information services: a platform for self-directed continuing medical education for front line decision makers *Postgraduate Medical Journal* 91:83–91.

O'CONNOR DAVIES, P. H. (1978) Medicines legislation and the ophthalmic optician. *Ophthalmic Optician, 18,* 688–694

O'CONNOR DAVIES, P. H. (1980) The use of ophthalmic drugs in the UK. *American Journal of Optometry and Physiological Optics, 57,* 925–926

OFFICE OF FAIR TRADING (1982) Opticians and Competition, HMSO, London

O'Sullivan, D (2020) Developing community eye care: the evolution of Wales' eye care services *EYE NEWS* 26 ISSUE 6 APRIL/MAY 2020 https://www.eyenews.uk.com/features/optometry/post/developing-community-eye-care-the-evolution-of-wales-eye-care-services

REDMOND, P. W. D. (1970) General Principles of English Law, Macdonald & Evans, London

SEATON, C. N. (1966) Aspects of the National Health Service Acts, Pergamon Press, Oxford

SIMMONDS, A. B. (1981) The attitude of the public towards the optometric profession. *Optician, 181,* June 26, 22–28

TAYLOR, S. P. (1982) Ophthalmic law. *Optician, 188,* No. 4757, 10

TAYLOR, S. P. (1983) New York State optometry: its legislation and practice. *Optician, 186,* No. 4820, 11–12

TAYLOR, S. P. (1984) Advertising — a professional spectacle. *Optician, 187,* No. 4930, 10–13

TAYLOR, S. P. (1986) The Effect of the Health and Social Security Act 1988 on the Profession of Optometry in the UK. *American Journal of Optometry and Physiological Optics* 63, 377–381

TAYLOR, S. P. (1991) The Opticians Act 1989 and UK Optometry. *Ophthalmic and Physiological Optics,* 11, 185–190

TAYLOR, S. P. (1991) The OSAC and UK Optometry. *Ophthalmic and Physiological Optics,* 11, 271–274

TAYLOR S. P. (1998) The Negligent Professional *Optician 216* No 5682 26–27

TAYLOR S. P. & EDWARDS K. H. (1999) Fitness to Practise Procedure *Optician, 217,* No 5685, 32–34

TAYLOR S. P. (2002) Law in Optometric Practice Butterworth Heinemann

WALDING, N. and LAUNDY, P. (1961) An Encyclopaedia of Parliament. Cassell, London

WARBURTON T (2013) Testing Retest Interval Times Optometry *Today* 17/5/2013 p 36–39

WISSE R. P. L, MUIJZER M. B, CASSANO F, GODERFROOIJ D. A, PREVO Y. F. D. M, SOETERS N (2019) Validation of an Independent Web-Based Tool for Measuring Visual Acuity and Refractive Error (the Manifest versus Online Refractive Evaluation Trial): Prospective Open-Label Noninferiority Clinical Trial. *J Med Internet Res* 2019;21(11):e14808 doi: 10.2196/14808

YARMOCSKY, R. (1984) The legal diversification of optometry. *Journal of the American Optometric Association,* 55, 665–669.

Reports

Report of the Committee appointed by the Minister of Health and the Secretary of State for Scotland on the Optical Practitioners (Registration) Bill 1927: Cmnd 2999, HMSO, London (December 1927)

Report of the Eye Services Committee to the Ophthalmic Sub-committee of the Negotiating Committee of the Medical Profession and the Joint Emergency Committee of the Optical Profession: Ministry of Health (May 1947)

Report of the Interdepartmental Committee on the Statutory Registration of Opticians: Cmnd 8531, HMSO, London (April 1952)

Price Commission report on prices of private spectacles and contact lenses: Report No. 20, HMSO, London (August 1976)

Opticians and Competition HMSO, London: (December 1982)

Primary Health Care, an agenda for discussion: Cmnd 9771, HMSO, London (1986)

The Government's Competition Policies and Optometry — London, Association of Optometrists (1987)

The Future of the Profession of Optometry — London British College of Optometrists (1989)

Report of the review of optical services undertaken by the Optical Services Audit Committee — London, General Optical Council (1990)

Vision for Optics in 2000. Henley Centre (1990)

Review of Prescribing, Supply and Administration of Medicines Part 1 (1998)

Review of Prescribing, Supply and Administration of Medicines Final Report (1999)

Optics at a Glance Series FODO (1985 to 2014)

'Trust Assurance and Safety': *the regulation of health professionals in the 21st century* (2007)

'Enabling Excellence: Autonomy and Accountability for Health and Social Care Staff' (2011) at http://www.nice.org.uk/guidance/mpg2/resources

Foresight Project Report 2020health (2016)

Community Eye Care Services: Review (Scotland) (2017)

Professional/Government Publications

Association of British Dispensing Opticians (2019) Advice and Guidelines

AOP (1999) Starting an Optometric Practice

AOP (1999) The Eye examination and related matters

British Standard (2004 & 2008) BS 2738-3:2004+A1:2008 Spectacle lenses Specification for the presentation of prescriptions and prescription orders for ophthalmic lenses

British Standard (2011) BS EN ISO 8624:2011 (Ophthalmic Optics. Spectacle Frames. Measuring System and Terminology)

British Standard (2017) BS EN ISO 21987:2017 — Ophthalmic optics — Mounted lenses.

Clinical Governance toolkits (England and Wales)

College of Optometrists (1999) Primary Eye Care Services

College of Optometrists (2001) Clinical Audit Framework for Optometric Practice

College of Optometrists (2002) Code of ethics and guidance for professional conduct

College of Optometrists (2021) Guidance for Professional Practice

College of Optometrists (2021) Optometrists Formulary

College of Optometrists (2021) Clinical Management Guidelines

College of Physicians and Surgeons of Nova Scotia and College of Registered Nurses of Nova Scotia (2005) *Guidelines for Delegated Medical Functions & Medical Directives*

Department of Health (1997) FPN 706 — GOS

Department of Health (1997) FPN713 — Advice and Clarification of General Ophthalmic Services (GOS) Procedures

Department of Health (1997) "The New NHS"

Department of Health (1998) "A First-Class Service"

Department of Health (2000) "The NHS Plan"

Department of Health. "Memorandum of Understanding — Frequency of GOS Sight Tests" (2002)

Dorset Health Authority (1999) Early testing criteria

Eye Health Examination Wales Services manual (2018) http://www.eyecare.wales.nhs.uk/document/328468

FODO (2021) Website https://www.fodo.com

GOC/AOP (2017) *Do you know the law on selling contact lenses?*

GOC (2021) Consultation feedback on CPD https://consultation.optical.org/standards-and-cet/cetreview/

GOC guidance for case examiners: https://goc.pixl8.london/download.cfm?docid=445A5485-0F1E-4410-AC5F7C8C7C9D6638

GOC Guidance for the Investigating Committee https://optical.org/media/zotjadhh/investigation-committee-guidance.pdf

GOC (2016) Standards of Practice for Optometrists and Dispensing Opticians https://standards.optical.org/the-standards/optometrists-and-dispensing-opticians/.

GOC (2022) Illegal Practice Protocol

Health Services Circular 1999/051 GOS increases in Spectacle Voucher Values, changes in definitions

NHS England (2021) Advice on content of a sight test

NHS England (2018) General Ophthalmic Mandatory Services Model Contract — Gateway reference: 08309

NHS Executive (1996) "Complaints — Guidance pack for optometrists"

NHS Executive (1996) "Primary Care: The Future"

NHS Executive (2000) "Action on Cataracts"

NHS Executive (2001) "Optical Point of Service checks in England"

NHS UK — Clinical Investigation — NHS Data Dictionary — *datadictionary. nhs.uk* › nhs_business_definitions › clinical investigation

NIEN — Northern Ireland Eyecare Network (2021) http://www.hscboard.hscni. net/our-work/integrated-care/ophthalmic-services/

NHS Wales (2021) Wales Eye Care Services, Wales. http://www.eyecare.wales. nhs.uk/home

Optical Confederation (2009) Clinical Governance Toolkit — QUALITY IN OPTOMETRY — Second Domain: Clinical Outcomes

Optical confederation (2012) Guidance on Social Media and Electronic Communication

Optical Confederation (2013) Clinical consensus panel report on the use of fluorescein in primary care.

Optical Confederation (2022) Making Accurate Claims

Optical Confederation. (2014) Template documents for complaints

Optical Confederation. (2014) Template documents for Freedom of Information Requests

Pocket Oxford Dictionary (1992) Oxford University Press

Quality in Optometry Toolkit https://www.qualityinoptometry.co.uk/

Scottish eyecare services: Review 2017 https://www.gov.scot/publications/ community-eyecare-services-review/

Index

Printed in the United States
by Baker & Taylor Publisher Services